YOU
PROMISED
TO DO
NO HARM

YOU PROMISED

A TRUE STORY OF LOVE, LOSS, AND THE HORROR OF HEALTHCARE DISPARITY FOR ONE AFRICAN-AMERICAN FAMILY

TO DO NO HARM

Jonnie Ramsey Brown, MBA, CPA, CISA

All names of individuals and institutions have been changed for privacy, except those used with permission.

In memory of Thomas James Brown

My Husband, my Baby

To Baby,

Thank you for spending your life with me

Thank you for loving me when I didn't even know

That love is what I needed most

Thank you for choosing me

A perfect gentleman, such a gentle man

You told me, "Remember who loves you"

So, when I think of you

What comes to mind most is how much you loved me

What did I do to deserve to be loved like this?

I promise you

For as long as I have breath

Others will know you

And will know what happened to you

Losing you has given me a new purpose

I love you, Baby

I love you with all my heart

You told me, "You're mine"

Yes, I'm yours, Baby

For the rest of my life

I will always belong to you

From Your Baby

CONTENTS

INTRODUCTION

THE DOCTORS' PROMISE

EVERYONE WHO KNEW THOMAS AND ME RECOGNIZED THAT WE were soulmates.

Our unconditional love and mutual respect were at the forefront of our relationship twenty-four hours a day. If there ever was a disagreement, especially in the latter portion of our forty-five years together, it was always about each of us wanting to concede—to get along with the other. We were best friends.

Thomas lived, it seemed, to love me and please me. I felt so secure with him, and I could always be myself because he completely understood and appreciated me. Although intellectually I knew that we all must leave this world one day, I never thought about life without him. It never occurred to me that that day would come much sooner than I had ever imagined.

* * *

I will never get over what happened to my husband in that Florida hospital in 2017. The hospital failed us in so many ways. Not only did they fail to provide the standard of care required for his condition, but they also did not even bother to show a modicum of compassion or concern for his well-being—or mine, for that matter.

I wanted so badly to believe that doctors embraced the Hippocratic oath, a pledge to refrain from causing harm or hurt. This ethical code has been adopted as a guide of conduct by the medical profession throughout the ages and is still used in graduation ceremonies at most medical schools.

The Hippocratic oath has evolved over time and is updated regularly by national medical associations to keep up with changing times. It now states that overtreatment must be avoided and that warmth, sympathy, and understanding may outweigh the surgeon's knife or the chemist's drug. It also states that physicians should not be ashamed to say, "I know not" and call upon their colleagues when the skills of another are needed for patient recovery. Physicians will remember that they do not treat a fever chart or a cancerous growth, but a sick human being, whose illness may affect the person's family and economic stability. Responsibilities include these related problems, if they are to care adequately for the sick.

Above all, the oath emphasizes: do no harm.

I had read and heard stories about the disparity in healthcare for African Americans in the United States, but fortunately, Thomas and I had never experienced it before. And why should we? We had the best health insurance available and selected our healthcare providers carefully.

It was surreal for me to leave Florida without my husband by my side. It was just too much to bear. The only way I found to deal with what happened there was to fight for him and his memory for the rest of my life—to bring awareness and change to a system that allowed this to happen.

Thomas told me that I often fool others because I appear to be a mild-mannered, easygoing person. People, he said, simply have no idea what they are up against when I decide to take on a cause. This book represents my cause.

* * *

As I started writing this book in 2020, detailing our fairy-tale romance and how our lives were forever altered by those medical professionals who violated their oath, I saw the horrific murder of George Floyd on the news. I saw him step out of his car, knowing that he was in trouble. I saw him try to be respectful, hoping that would change the outcome. I saw how he was killed by those who promise to "protect and serve," just as Thomas was killed by those who promise to "do no harm."

One happened on a public street where people could pull out their cameras, while the other happened privately behind hospital walls, but these horrific acts occur everywhere, every day. Actual and unconscious biases are real and can affect decision-making and behaviors. Just as law enforcement is being forced to confront the reality that African Americans are being harmed unnecessarily, the medical profession must come to terms with the fact that they also play a role in hurting people of color.

My husband did not have to die.

My life did not have to be shattered.

Real people and their families are affected by the neglectful acts of those in the medical profession who we seek out for help.

Thomas taught me how to fight for our relationship with the same intensity that he did, and I am still fighting for him. It is my hope that after people read this book, the movement grows to seriously identify, address, and rectify healthcare disparity for people of color in the United States.

Academia and governmental agencies are developing strategies to address the issue. It is encouraging that students at some medical schools have added to the oath their pledge to fight racial injustice and misinformation. Still, patients and families must do their part as well. Whether it is obtaining a healthcare advocate to navigate the healthcare system and treatment options, or formally complaining to hospital accreditation commissions, or filing complaints with state medical oversight boards, or filing a lawsuit in court, or advocating for legislation, we must work together quickly to create a new environment within the medical profession where consequences await those who hurt us—those who promised to do no harm.

PART I

THE LIFE

CHAPTER 1

A GENTLEMAN—AND A GENTLE MAN

THOMAS SHOULD HAVE WALKED AWAY FROM ME THE FIRST TIME we met.

I am so fortunate he did not.

He arrived at a time in my life when I was angry at every man that came my way. My first marriage was abusive, and I carried a great deal of trauma from it. As such, the few relationships I found myself in after my divorce did not work out either. In fact, one of those men told me that I did not need a man. That I could take care of myself.

And he was right.

The truth was that every man I had met seemed to be looking for a weak-willed, helpless woman who depended on a man for her very existence or—worse yet—a woman who would do anything it took to keep a man. I am neither woman.

So, I decided to be by myself for a while. I focused on me, my lovely son from that first marriage, and my pursuit of the education that had eluded me due to the difficulties I faced before and during that abusive relationship.

One evening in 1972, a remarkable gentleman changed all of that.

* * *

My friend Joanne called that night and asked if I would go with her to a nightclub after work. It was a spot on Crenshaw and Century Boulevards in Inglewood, California, called The Name of the Game.

I love that name, I thought.

I was twenty-three years old, and although I loved to dance, nightclubs were not really my favorite place to be. Besides, I did not drink, and just about every club had a two-drink minimum.

"I don't really feel like going," I said.

"I always go with *you* when you want to go somewhere," Joanne said. "Look, I'll even buy your drinks. Okay?"

When she sensed I still was not quite convinced, she went on to tell me that she was meeting a guy there and she needed me. If she liked him, she would leave with him, but if she was not feeling him, then she would tell him she was with me.

My four-year-old son, Michael, was already staying with my parents since I would be on the late shift that evening, and I eventually warmed up to the idea that it would be nice to get out afterward. So, with a begrudging smile, I agreed. Joanne was happy and told me she would pick me up on her way, as my house was closest to the club.

After work, I put on a purple pair of stretch hip-huggers that rode low on the hips and flared out from the knee into bell bottoms, with a long-sleeved purple leotard to match. I did not put on any makeup, except for a little bit of lipstick, and only wore a touch of perfume, as I sometimes have an allergic reaction to makeup and fragrances.

That night, I decided to don a soft-brown Afro wig. I rarely wore wigs, but it was the perfect time to give this one a try, as I was not looking to meet or impress anyone. Large Afros were the latest craze, and if I was going to the club, I was going to do it right. A pair of large, gold-tone hoop earrings set the whole outfit off.

Joanne might have been the one looking for a man, but she was not going to show me up.

When we arrived at the club, we were ushered to two tables that, pushed together, sat eight people. Joanne and I sat on the far side next to each other, facing the crowd, listening to the live band. The lead singer had a fantastic voice and belted out all the hits:

The Temptations' "Just My Imagination."

Marvin Gaye's "What's Going On."

The Isley Brothers' "It's Your Thing."

Al Green's "Let's Stay Together."

Gladys Knight's "If I Were Your Woman."

The Isley Brothers' "Love the One You're With."

Looking back, it seems even the band knew what was destined to happen that night.

Joanne ordered our drinks, and before too long, her "date" arrived, a young brother named Melvin. She introduced us, and Melvin sat on the other side of Joanne so that she was between the two of us. The two of them started talking and quickly lost interest in me.

Elbow on the table, I rested my chin on the back of my hand, terribly bored, occasionally rolling my eyes at the game Melvin was running on Joanne. At least, the game he *thought* he was running on Joanne.

The club was a favorite hangout for folks on that side of town, and the place filled up fast. It got so crowded that they were running out of seating, and a very handsome man was ushered over to where we sat. He took a seat at the head of the table next to me.

He was tall with long legs and dressed sharply in a sweater, slacks, and above-the-ankle boots that zipped up on the inside ankle—a staple of men's shoes during the seventies. He was also fair-complected with a mustache, long sideburns, and the biggest Afro I had seen outside of the movies or the entertainment industry.

That hair. My goodness, that hair. He had pulled some of the curls in the front down onto his forehead, creating a "V" shape. That Afro had so much body, he could have starred in a shampoo commercial for healthy, bouncy hair. Every time he moved his head, that Afro swayed right along with him.

Better than all of that were his eyes. Beautiful, hazel, and mesmerizing. The creases around those eyes made them smile all on their own, and though I did not want to admit it, they put me quickly at ease. It was hard not to stare at his every move as he ordered his two drinks. He put his money on the table, and while waiting for the waitress to return, he turned his attention to me.

Captivated as I was, I was not interested in him.

Here I was, a young divorcée with enough experience in my short life to know that he was not someone I wanted to get mixed up with. A player like him probably had a woman for every night of the week and even more women waiting for their chance. He was the kind of handsome that would make other women bold enough to flirt with him in front of the woman he was with.

Nope. I had no desire to get caught up in that kind of drama.

He caught me looking and stared steadily into my eyes. As he flashed a charming smile, I thought, *Oh no, you are just too smooth.*

"Hi," he said. "What's your name?"

I replied to his smile with an irritated look. After a long pause, I said, "Jonnie Marsh." Then I looked away in the opposite direction.

"My name is Thomas Brown," he said to the back of my head. "Nice meeting you."

I glanced back over my shoulder to see that his drinks had arrived. Once again, he caught me watching as he smiled and took a sip.

"Would you like a drink?" he asked.

I stared at the two drinks sitting in front of me, then looked him squarely in his eyes, and said, with no small amount of rudeness, "Can't you see I have two drinks already?"

Despite my tone, he did not flinch—just intensely stared at me and smiled. He continued to make small talk, smiling pleasantly the whole time. His eyes and his deep voice were so kind that I found it difficult to continue being rude.

We talked about the music the band played and what part of town we lived in. We discovered that we had attended the same high school and that we were both currently attending college part-time in the evenings. He told me he spent four years in the military, serving the country during the Vietnam conflict, and I respected him for that, having lost many of my high school classmates to the war.

Then he asked me what I did for a living.

I *hated* that question. When men posed it, I had reason to assume they wanted to know if I had a good job making good money so that they could get their hands on it. Thomas asking me that was all it took for my unpleasant self to reemerge.

"If I told you, you probably wouldn't even understand."

He laughed. "I think I'll understand. Try me. I'm curious."

I hesitated for a few moments. "I'm an air traffic controller."

"Oh, I understand. I was in the Air Force. I fully comprehend what you do."

I heard respect in his voice, and I appreciated that. Then, the band broke into a slow song, a cover of "I Don't Want to Do Wrong" by Gladys Knight and the Pips, and Thomas stood up and held out his hand.

"Would you like to dance?"

I shrugged, giving him my hand. He took my hand in his, so gently, and escorted me to the dance floor.

Now, I know what you might be thinking. How did I go from "Don't you see I have two drinks?" to a slow drag on the dance floor? First of all, that Old Spice he had on was just the right amount. Secondly, I will remind you that while I did not drink, I *did* dance, though I would not dance with just anyone. Thomas appeared to be a gentleman, and I did not mind dancing with someone who was respectful.

Out on the dance floor, I liked the way I fit in Thomas's arms. He was tall and strong, but gentle when he put his arms around me. Still, there was a part of me that wanted to mess with his mind a little bit. He was good looking, and he knew it, and I was supposed to be impressed by that. So, I pressed myself up against him, grinding to the music, giving him the impression that I liked dancing with him. That is how we slow danced back in the 1970s.

Let us just say I came to the conclusion that he liked dancing with me too—but I would be leaving soon, with or without Joanne, and I had no interest in pursuing this encounter any further.

The song ended and we returned to the table. Joanne must have had enough of Melvin, because she was ready to go. *Good*, I thought, *I'm ready to get out of here.* I told Thomas I would see him again sometime, and Joanne I left the club and headed for her car.

We did not leave right away, because Joanne had to give me the rundown on Melvin. As she broke down exactly why he just was not her type, I heard a tap on my window and turned to see Thomas standing there. I rolled down the window and glared at him.

"I'd like to get your telephone number so I can call you later."

"I don't give out my number," I snapped. Then something in me relented, and I added, "But give me yours and maybe I'll call you."

My reaction wasn't much about Thomas. Since I had decided to take a hiatus from relationships with men, I did not want men I had just met calling my house. But that did not stop me from calling them and seeing if they wanted to take me to dinner. The truth was, I did not cook and had no desire to learn, but I enjoyed having company when going out to eat. I could see myself letting Thomas buy me a meal.

Once Joanne dropped me off at home, I put his number in my phone book.

* * *

A few weeks later, I decided that I wanted to break the monotony and eat a nice meal at a nice restaurant. I would usually buy food to-go from a local restaurant or McDonald's for me and Michael, or we would go to my parents' house, where my mother always had plenty of food and we were always welcomed.

I pulled out my phone book and started at the beginning of the alphabet to find myself a dinner date. When no one in the A's piqued my interest, I moved on to the B's and came across Thomas Brown—that good-looking guy from The Name of the Game. He seemed nice enough. Surprisingly so.

I called him up.

"This is Jonnie Marsh. Do you remember me?"

"Yes, I remember you."

"Do you want to take me to dinner?"

No need for chitchat. I just wanted a simple yes or no so I could get on with finding a willing date.

Thomas said yes, and we made a date for that upcoming Friday night. He said he would pick me up and asked for my phone number in case there was a change in plans. This time, I gave it to him—and a good thing too. Two hours before he was due to pick me up, my phone rang.

"I have a problem," Thomas said.

"Oh? What's *your* problem?" I asked, with no small amount of attitude. At that time, I felt like all men had problems—and in that moment, Thomas was no different than any other man. I was annoyed because I had already dropped Michael off at my parents' home and arranged for him to spend the night so that I would not have to wake them later.

"So, my money is kinda funny, and I have to pay rent this week. We can go to a restaurant, but that would pretty much be it for the evening. Or I can cook for you, and then we can go out afterward."

I thought about it for a moment. I did call him unexpectedly, and I did not want to cause a problem. So, I said, rudely, "You cook for me."

"Sure, no problem," he said. I could not help but notice that no matter what I said or how impolite I was when I said it, Thomas always maintained his composure. He never reacted to my negativity.

It turned out to be one of his finest and most consistent qualities.

After we hung up, I put on a short black dress and a short dress jacket. The dress hit just above my knees, with black pantyhose and black heels to complement it, but I did not wear the wig that I had worn the first time we met.

Thomas arrived right on time, just like a military man would, dressed as sharply as the day he approached me at the club. I asked him to take a seat while I finished getting ready. When I returned, he said, "What happened to your Afro?"

"Oh, that was a wig. I usually wear my hair straightened like this. That night I met you was actually the first time I wore that wig. Does it make a difference?"

"No, not at all," he said, laughing. "I thought that was your hair. I was just expecting something else."

Well, that kind of ticked me off, but I told myself I really did not care what he thought anyway. *Just feed me like you promised me you would do,* I thought.

Outside, Thomas opened and closed the passenger door to his green Pinto for me. He drove off to where he lived in Baldwin Hills, a desirable area in Los Angeles. Thomas told me he did not care much for the Pinto, and that his favorite car was one he owned while he was in high school and in the military—a 1955 metallic green Chevy.

"I saved my money from a part-time job I had in high school," he said. "My father owned a garage at the time and told me he had found the perfect car for me. He even went ahead and bought it with my money without telling me. But it needed lots of bodywork and repairs. I was so disappointed when I first saw that car, until my father, a couple of his friends, and I worked on it and brought it to pristine condition. Man, that car was so sharp."

"Where is it now?"

His face dropped. "My brother wrecked it while I was away in the service."

Thomas talked about how everyone in high school knew about him and his sharp car, and he would often give rides to classmates. Back in the day, in the early sixties, very few students had their own cars.

There were whole family households that did not have cars, so I could sense that Thomas was proud to have worked and paid for his car himself.

We arrived at his building and entered his small apartment, where music was already playing at a low volume. Thomas gestured toward a blue velvet couch, where I had a seat and took in the feel of the place. He kept it neat and clean. There was a heavy coffee table in the center of the living room and two end tables with marble inlays and lamps that lent ambiance to the room.

"May I get you a drink?" Thomas asked.

"I don't drink. 7UP is fine, if you have it. Thank you." I looked over to the dining room to see that Thomas had taken the time to formally set the table with a bouquet of fresh flowers as the centerpiece. He returned from the kitchen with drinks and sat down next to me on the couch.

"I'm glad you let me make dinner," he said. "I love to cook. Dinner will be ready shortly, but we can relax in the meantime." He reached into the compartment in the coffee table. "Do you mind if I show you some pictures that were taken while I was in the Air Force? I was stationed in some interesting places around the world."

I agreed, and Thomas flashed an eager smile. He flipped through the pages of a photo album as we looked at photos from the Philippines and Vietnam. He talked about how he had almost made a career of the Air Force and how, if he had a chance to do it over again, he would re-enlist.

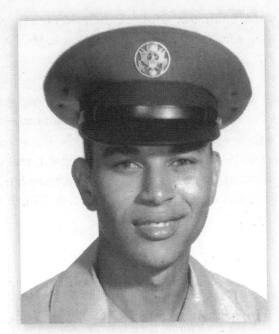

Airman Thomas J. Brown.
United States Air Force. About 1961

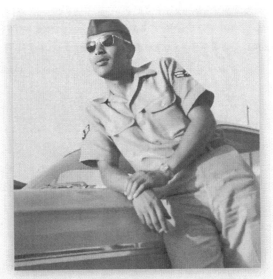

Airman First Class Thomas J. Brown. About 1963

After about twenty minutes, Thomas excused himself to check on dinner. When dinner was ready, he invited me into the dining room. I picked up our drinks and headed in that direction.

The table setting was even more impressive than I had first thought. A white linen tablecloth covered the table. Thomas had neatly placed folded cloth napkins on dinner plates that were sitting on oversized decorative plates. The silverware was formally set, and there were water goblets on the table. A bread basket sat in the middle, lined with a cloth napkin folded over warm rolls. A butter knife and two pats of butter were on each dinner roll plate.

He gestured to where he wanted me to sit.

Thomas took the dinner plates from the table and returned with a feast on them—T-bone steak, baked potato with the works, and baby asparagus. I was so impressed as I waited for him to sit down and indicate what I should do next. He sat at the head of the table, placing his napkin in his lap in a very cultured manner, and I followed suit. Then he raised his glass for a toast, and I did the same.

"Cheers," he said.

"Cheers."

The steak was delicious—tender and so well seasoned—and I told him so. "Where did you learn to cook?"

"My parents and my mother's family taught me how. My mother's sister, Aunt Anna, was a dietician and worked for a wealthy white family in Abbeville, South Carolina. I would visit them in the summers when I was a kid. She taught me not just about cooking, but also the proper presentation of food. That woman could make a simple peanut butter and jelly sandwich look and taste amazing."

"Well, I know nothing about cooking," I said, a little embarrassed. "My mother always took care of the meals because she enjoyed it too. She sometimes asked us to snap beans or shuck corn, and we definitely had to do the dishes, but she pretty much took care of the rest."

"And my father told me to never depend on a woman for my food," he said, flashing a charming smile.

I studied his face to see if he was ragging on me. I saw no judgment in those smiling eyes. Just teasing and playfulness.

* * *

I would later learn that the way Thomas set the table, the way he put the napkin in his lap, and the way he treated me—all of it went against all of the perceptions I had formed about him. It turned out that the cooking, the table setting, and his calm and gentle manner stemmed from his mother's influence.

Thomas's mother was a proud but quiet woman, and her well-to-do, multiracial family was relatively well known in Abbeville. Most of them were light-skinned, looking more white than Black, and Thomas was no exception. He had those hazel eyes and that pretty hair.

Thomas's father was very handsome as well, often photographed in three-piece suits, the epitome of cool. It was easy to see how Mrs. Brown had fallen for him.

However, Mrs. Brown's family did not approve of her marrying him because he was not of their stature and he could not provide her with the lifestyle she had known all of her life. Mr. Brown eventually was employed as a Pullman porter, a coveted job during the heyday of passenger trains, which required him to work long hours away from home. The job was based out of Chicago, so Thomas grew up in the Ida B. Wells projects on Chicago's South Side. At the time, of all the projects, it was the place to be because it was one of the newer ones—but it was the projects, nonetheless. Because of this, Thomas's family were outcasts among his mother's people.

Sadly, Mr. Brown was a player and was not faithful to Mrs. Brown, resulting in her threatening to leave him on more than one occasion. She had talks with Thomas, who was the youngest of her four children, and he saw how hurt she was by his father's actions.

These talks would become defining moments in Thomas's life. He was closest to his mother and saw the dynamics between her and his father. He grew up vowing he would never treat his future wife in that manner—that she would come first in his life and would always feel secure in their relationship.

I can testify that Thomas kept his commitment to do just that.

* * *

We finished dessert—a pie that Thomas humbly admitted he did not bake—and I told Thomas that the meal was fantastic. "Never did I imagine I'd be getting a private dinner tonight."

"I'm glad you liked it. I enjoyed watching you enjoy it," he said. Those were the words of a true chef. He took great pleasure in cooking, but perhaps even more so in watching others enjoy his food.

After I turned down his offer for coffee, he told me he wanted to take me to a nightclub not too far from his apartment. I agreed, and once again, he opened and closed my car door for me. He assumed that because we met at the club that going out to them was something I liked to do. It was not, but I had agreed to dinner and going out afterwards. Besides, he appeared to have such a kind soul and I was enjoying his company, so I did not mind the evening continuing.

I was not familiar with the club he had chosen. When we walked in, Thomas looked around for a moment until he spotted his two friends at a table across the room. He placed his hand on the small of my back and guided me to the table to introduce me to Charles and Earl. They were polite enough, but quickly returned to their own conversation, laughing and essentially ignoring the two of us. That annoyed me and made me feel like just another one of Thomas's women I imagined he kept around.

I had to remind myself that this was just a dinner arrangement and nothing more.

We were at the club for about an hour. Thomas had a few drinks while I drank 7UP. I asked him what year he graduated from our high school. Turned out it was the same year my sister and her best friend graduated, though I did not tell him that at the time. *Oh, I'm going to have to ask my sister about him*, I thought.

As nice a time as we were having, I figured at the end of the night, Thomas was going to take me home and that would be it. But that line of thinking did not last. When we returned to my house, I asked if he would like to come inside for a few minutes, and he agreed. I had surprised myself that I wanted him to, but he had been so nice, completely shattering all the expectations I had of him. I loved talking to Thomas, and it seemed he felt the same. He was just so different from all the other men I had dated—so much kinder and more mature.

We sat in my living room and talked for hours about our lives. We discovered that we had both been married before. Where I had a son, he had a daughter, with my son being older by one year. I confessed to him that I was married for less than two years because it was such a bad situation—so much so that I did not ever want to get married again. I told him how I had tried to keep my marriage intact, but that my husband was not a nice man and would not keep a job, and that it was not a marriage worth saving. I had been through more than he wanted to know.

Then I asked him what happened in his marriage.

"I'm still married," Thomas said.

Disgusted, I slowly shook my head and sucked my teeth. "Then what are you doing here with me?"

"It's not like that. My wife left me under the pretense of going on a vacation to visit her family in Louisiana." Thomas looked directly at me when he said it, and the pain in his eyes was as clear as the words he spoke. "She called to tell me she was staying a little longer and asked for some money, which I sent. Then she called again, wanting to stay longer, wanting more money. Finally, I asked her how this vacation was affecting her job here in Los Angeles.

"That's when she told me she had quit her job some time ago. This whole vacation thing was a sham. She basically quit her job and left me. Things were not good between us, and we didn't communicate all that well, so in all honesty, it was a good thing. We had actually broken up not too long after we met, but two months later, she called to tell me she was pregnant. I wanted to do the right thing by her, but we really didn't get along very well from the beginning. There is more to this story, but she went back to Louisiana, and that's where she is now."

I was curious. "Do you think you and your wife will get back together?"

"I don't think so, no. She's close to her family and wants to live in Louisiana. She wants me to transfer to Baton Rouge on my job, but I'm not going to do that. There's little communication and little trust. I don't think we can make it. It's best that she stays in Louisiana. Truthfully, I'm more concerned about my daughter because I don't get a chance to see her as much as I would like."

Before we knew it, daylight peeked out from under the blinds on my windows. It was after six o'clock in the morning. Though I wanted to continue the conversation, I just could not. I was exhausted.

"I'm so sleepy," I said, yawning. "I don't think I can stay awake much longer. It's so late—or rather early. Do you want to go to bed?"

Now I know how that sounds—but do not rush to judgment.

Thomas followed me to my bedroom. I slipped out of my clothes and climbed into bed in my underwear, and Thomas did the same. I turned on my side to look at him for a few moments.

"Thomas, I don't want to...do anything. It's difficult turning over to someone new."

"I understand," he said.

We lay there for a few minutes, and then I fell asleep.

* * *

About six months into our relationship, I asked Thomas why he pursued me when I had been so mean and rude to him.

"I thought you were an intelligent young lady. So cute with so much on the ball. But I couldn't understand why you were so unhappy. And you didn't behave like most of the women I meet in the club, throwing themselves at me and making every suggestive comment you could imagine. Believe it or not, I don't really appreciate that. I could see in your eyes that I didn't impress you, and I liked that. And just so you know—I knew you were going to call me."

"And how did you know that?" I asked with a sly smile.

"Because I'm a nice fella." He grinned. "Also, I wasn't arbitrarily seated at your table at The Name of the Game. I specifically asked to be seated next to you."

As sweet as all that was, it struck me that Thomas recognized my pain from the moment he met me—but he also recognized that there was more to me than the sullen woman that I had first presented to him.

It did not take long to learn even more how deeply troubled Thomas was about the state of his own personal affairs. He had so much love to give and was looking for someone to pour all of his love into—someone who would love him back just as much. I think he truly believed that he could love me and heal me—and in the process, heal himself.

* * *

Thomas respected my wishes that first night. He eventually awoke first, pushing back the covers and sitting up on his side of the bed. His stirring woke me.

"Good morning," he said. "I'm leaving now. I'll call you later?"

"Sure."

He did call me later that day. He came by to see me again that evening.

Some kind of a connection existed between us that could not be denied.

That is why Thomas Brown—that gentleman and gentle man—never left my side again for the rest of his life.

CHAPTER 2

REMEMBER
WHO LOVES YOU

"Oh no. You've got to be kidding! Not him!"

That was my sister's reaction when I asked her if she remembered Thomas Brown.

"Well, what does that mean?" I asked.

"I remember that he was so annoying. He always wanted to play. He was always joking around and teasing everybody. He used to work my nerves."

"Is he a nice guy? How well did you know him?"

"He was nice, I guess," Tommie said.

My sister's name is Thomasine, but we call her Tommie for short. It was quite common in the South at one time for women to be named after males in the family, such as Bobbie, Frankie, and Willie, and even though my parents had moved from Toomsuba, Mississippi, to Detroit, they had kept the tradition alive.

"He had a car in high school and a bunch of us would pile into his car at lunchtime to get something to eat," Tommie continued. "Or to go to the beach or park. He sometimes hung out with Roland, whose brother Clarence was Mary's boyfriend for many years." Mary has been Tommie's best friend since childhood.

"Did any of you date Thomas?"

"Are you kidding? He was such a pest. He was relentless in his teasing. I never really saw him with a specific girl. Most of the times when I saw him, he was with a group of people acting crazy and clowning around."

The next time I spoke to Thomas, I told him that he probably knew my sister since they graduated high school together.

"Thomasine is your sister?" he said, laughing. "Yes, I remember her. Her best friend is Mary, right? Do you know her too?

"Yep, my sister and Mary are still close friends, and Mary is like a member of the family."

"Well, I'm looking forward to seeing Thomasine and Mary again. Tell them that for me."

When they did see each other again, I could see what Tommie was talking about. He began recalling memories from high school and immediately broke out into teasing, needling her to a point where she was getting aggravated. It was funny to watch this because, for the first time, I observed Thomas's outrageous playful side on full display.

* * *

I do not remember exactly when after that delightful dinner that Thomas started calling me "Baby"—but I know once he did, he never stopped. And neither did I.

The nickname meant so much to me—and still does to this day. No man had ever called me by any term of affection before. I loved it so much that I started calling him Baby too. We got to the point where just about every sentence of every conversation either started or ended with the word. We had gotten so silly about it that Tommie playfully told us we were just sick, and we would break down in fits of laughter.

It was not just an affectionate name though. Baby could also be a signal, depending on the inflection in our voices, to indicate whether or not one of us was getting annoyed with the other. And the times we called each other by our actual names? Watch out. That meant one of us was seriously upset, a situation where Baby just would not do, no matter what tone accompanied the word.

When I was on the receiving end of hearing my name, I would say, "Don't call me Jonnie."

"Well, that's your name, isn't it?" Thomas would say.

"No, it isn't."

"What is it then?"

"My name is Baby," I would say, smiling. We would both laugh, and whatever it was that had gotten us upset would almost always be forgotten.

Still, as with any couple, there were times when we could not laugh it away. When that happened, I refused to talk to him, should I say something that might get me in trouble. Though I knew in my heart that Thomas would never hurt me, my first husband had conditioned me to never push a man to a point where physical violence might be a consideration.

But it never came to that with Thomas.

When we were both quite upset, I would tell Thomas I was done talking and I would go to bed and turn on the TV. After a few hours, he would tiptoe into the bedroom, sit on the side of the bed, and ask if I was still angry—and we would talk.

He listened, always letting me have my say. He would tell me with no lie in those hazel eyes that he understood why I was upset, and then he would place a soft kiss on my lips. As much as I did not like to see him upset, I believe he could not handle my being mad at him for any amount of time at all. He worked so hard to please me and make me happy. He loved me that much—and I loved him the same way.

Imagine—the worst thing we ever called each other was by our given names.

* * *

"Women don't realize how much power they have," Thomas said out of the blue one day. By this time, I had asked Thomas to move in with me, and he was relaxing in the family room and sipping on his wine. I was sitting on the floor, working on one of the many projects I always had going on, with papers spread everywhere.

"What do you mean by that, Baby?" I asked.

"Well, there's the physical thing where men sometimes find it difficult to control their desires. But when a man finds the woman he truly loves, he'll do almost anything to please her and to hold on to her."

"Oh." I thought for a moment. "Do I have that kind of power?"

He took another sip of wine and laughed. "See what I mean, Baby? You have no idea."

I remember how I would delay putting gas in my car until the last possible moment. I hated going to the gas station, so I would often call Thomas when I was on my way home from work to warn him that he might need to see about me if I ran out of gas. After a few calls like that, he became impatient with me and said to just let him know when my car needed gas and he would get it for me.

And because he loved to cook, Thomas would prepare anything I wanted, whether I saw it in a magazine or ate it at a restaurant. His cooking was an expression of his love, and just like the first time he made dinner, his happiness came from me enjoying the food he prepared especially for me.

One of my favorite meals is a hamburger with grilled onions. Thomas could fix the best burger, and when it was ready, he would ask me to come to the table. Before he put the plate down in front of me, he would look me in my eyes, give me a kiss, and say, "You're mine." I loved the way he claimed me as his own.

Thomas approached lovemaking in the same way he approached cooking—his satisfaction was very much tied to mine.

Since I had never had a healthy relationship with a man in the past, I did not know what a close and loving relationship was. Thomas gave me full body massages, something new to me as I used to be ticklish almost everywhere on my body. I laugh when I think about that now, but back then, it did not seem to matter much because Thomas was very playful himself. We had fun together no matter what we were doing.

Over time, Thomas taught me all about real sexual intimacy. I finally experienced closeness and emotional connectedness with a man who loved me. And I loved Thomas for being patient with me as he showed me what a truly positive, safe, trusting, and intimate relationship was supposed to be.

Thomas and I loved R & B music, and at some point on any given day, the radio was on or an album was playing on the stereo. One day, Thomas asked me if I liked Anita Baker's song entitled "Giving You the Best That I Got." I was familiar with the song but had never really listened to the lyrics because they were difficult to understand when sung. I had studied classical piano for six years as a preteen and teenager, so I was often content to listen only to the musical arrangement. "You should love that song, Baby," Thomas said affectionately. "The songwriter had you in mind when that song was written. It's about the person you are and why I love you, Baby."

My heart melted when I read the lyrics to this beautiful love song. The lyrics are about a woman who has finally found someone who truly loves her, and she vows to give her all to the relationship, wondering what more she can do to show her gratefulness. It was true. I appreciated Thomas so much for loving me, and I tried to let him know every day how much I loved and cherished him for changing my life.

I recall how a friend, who had stayed with us for a few days, remarked how we had the most loving and respectful relationship she had ever seen between a man and woman. She knew a lot of couples, but none of them had a connection and tenderness like Thomas and I shared.

Since observing us, she has a clearer understanding of what she wants from a relationship.

I also recall how one of our neighbors teased Thomas by saying he was setting a high bar for the rest of the men in the neighborhood, not just by filling up my gas tank—which was huge for the ladies—but in setting the tone for the quality of a relationship. Thomas got a big kick out of knowing that other men and women noticed how much he loved me and all he did to care for me.

We did not care what anyone else said about our non-traditional relationship. Thomas cooked and helped me clean, I handled the bills, and we shared parental duties—and it worked for us. We were happy because we were doing the things in our relationship that we most enjoyed and that also played to our personal strengths.

Thomas was a romantic through and through, always looking for new ways to please me and show me that he appreciated me. He held nothing back. There was love in every little gesture, every day. He truly was an amazing man.

*   *   *

On several occasions, Thomas said to me, "You don't see all these men out here looking at you, do you?"

When Thomas said that, I thought he was trying to start something, because my ex-husband often said something similar when he was trying to start an argument. Back then, I would just play dumb. The last thing I wanted was to get into a fight because I never knew how bad things might get. That experience conditioned me to react the same way when Thomas asked.

"No, I don't see it," I told him.

But I had not anticipated Thomas's response.

"That's another thing I like about you," he said. "You're a good-looking woman and you don't even know men are out here looking at you. You don't think you're all that. You don't even notice."

Even though he liked that about me, I knew he was sometimes jealous and worried about other men approaching me. I was happy in our relationship and had never given any indication that I was interested in someone else, but Thomas would still get insecure sometimes.

So, on many occasions, if Thomas knew I was going to be gone all day or if I had to go out of town for work or to see my parents, he would stop me at the door. He would hold me tight and shower me with kisses. Then he would look me straight in my eyes with those hazel eyes of his and say, "Remember who loves you."

No matter how many times I heard it, it just blew me away. I had never felt that kind of affection before. On the few occasions that men did approach me, that phrase was the first thing that came into my head. I had a man at home who loved me and took care of me and completely fulfilled me emotionally. There was no way I was going to mess that up.

He knew that line worked on me, but the best part of it all was that he really meant it when he said it.

* * *

Thomas understood human psychology, and it did not take him long to figure out that I had experienced fear and emotional trauma during my first marriage. I had put up a lot of walls to mask my feelings and insecurities, but he saw right through them.

He understood because the failure of his first marriage had disturbed him as well. In my experience, there were not many men who would share how hurt they were when their relationships did not work out—or share their contribution to the situation. All too often it was, "the wife did this" or "the wife did that." But not Thomas. He was open and honest about his failings and how hurt he was that his wife abandoned him.

His daughter, Nichelle, would come stay with us during the summers and on other occasions, and though we were raising our kids and working and going to school together, I never asked Thomas about getting a divorce. I never asked about marriage either. I truly enjoyed what we had, taking it day by day at a point in our lives where we both needed love and support from someone else.

Despite his fear that it might all go away again, Thomas took a chance on me. Things did not have to work out the way they did between us: I might not have been receptive to this relationship, or, worse yet, I could have been the kind of woman to take advantage of it. But the fact that Thomas laid his heart out for me spoke to the kind of man he was. He felt that loving me was well worth the risk.

I testify to this day that Thomas was the one that kept us together, not me. I would have left two, three, four times—maybe more— over the course of our relationship, especially when I was younger. I was such a hothead, self-confident intellectually but with little confidence in my dealings with the opposite sex. Any time we had some kind of disagreement, I would run to the intellectual side of my brain, the one that shouted, *I can take care of myself! I don't need this.*

Still, any time there was the slightest amount of friction between us, Thomas would flip the situation on its head and say something conciliatory or sweet that would make everything okay. He would remind me that we had a good relationship that was too strong to throw away over some nonsense. He always returned my focus to what we had, and that always helped us work things out.

That is when he told me that I never needed to go to those bad places in my head ever again. That we were going to agree that we would make it no matter what. When anything happened, we were going to put all our energy into fixing it.

I remember looking at him in amazement as he told me that. In my mind, those were the things women usually say to hold things together because men find it difficult to express their feelings. Not so with Thomas. He had great faith that we would always be happy and that we could get through anything. Together.

CHAPTER 3

LOVE BROUGHT US TOGETHER

WHEN WE FIRST MET, THOMAS WAS WORKING DURING THE DAY and going to junior college part-time. I wanted him to transfer to California State University, Los Angeles, where I was in attendance, but he was not sure if he had the right number of credits to do so. I asked him to get his transcripts so I could see if in fact he had enough credits—and he did. Thomas did not know that he was entitled to an additional sixteen general credits for the four years he had served in the military.

He was excited like a child when he got the acceptance letter. He could not thank me enough for encouraging me and making this happen. We tried to schedule our classes on the same evenings since we both worked during the day, always looking for ways to maximize our time together.

Back in 1970, I passed a test to become an air traffic controller after reading a recruitment flier on the bulletin board while working at the

US Post Office. The Federal Aviation Administration (FAA) was hiring women and minorities due to Affirmative Action, so I took advantage of the opportunity. At the same time, I continued to attend college part-time in the evenings for my accounting degree.

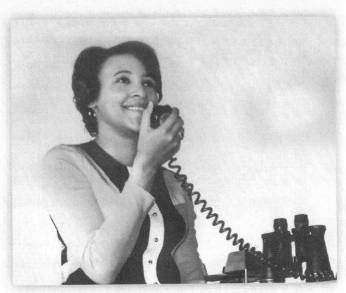

Jonnie, Air Traffic Controller. Santa Monica Tower.
Santa Monica, CA. About 1973

In early 1974, I realized that if I went to college full-time, I could finish my degree in nine months. When I told my supervisor at the FAA that I needed to quit to finish my degree, he said, "We're going to give you a leave of absence. You're not resigning." Being one of the first female and Black air traffic controllers, they did not want to lose me. So I did not turn down their offer, knowing that I had the option to return at any time, if I wanted to. Meanwhile, Thomas quit his job and made use of the G.I. Bill to go to college full-time as well. We both graduated at basically the same time—me in December 1974 and Thomas in September 1975.

We marched together in June 1975 to receive our diplomas. Thomas was allowed to march the quarter prior to finishing his program, rather than waiting nine months until the following June. I can still recall how incredible that day felt just as powerfully as I could back then.

In the photo of us standing together in our caps and gowns, Thomas's hand was on his chest, and he beamed with pride. His parents had attended the ceremony, and I saw in his eyes just how much it meant to him—it nearly brought him to tears. Thomas told me that his parents had never come to any events in his life, so that they were there for his graduation was a truly special time for him.

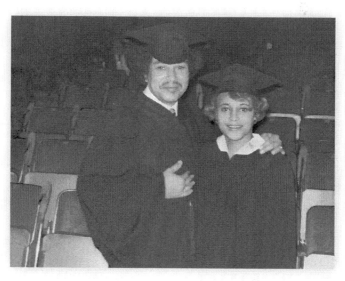

Thomas & Jonnie. College graduation.
California State University, Los Angeles. June 1975

I was equally proud—Thomas and I were both the first ones in our families to acquire a college education. Our parents grew up in the South during the height of Jim Crow laws and the Ku Klux Klan, and they struggled to partake in a system that did not provide the level of education afforded to the white children. Mine would tell me how a free education for Black children was only available through the eighth grade and how they would literally walk miles to and from school while the white kids were picked up by bus.

My father also told me that a high school education had to be paid for and required a move to a larger city. He was fortunate enough to complete eleventh grade, but circumstances derailed his plans to acquire his high school diploma. He was working for a white family in Meridian, Mississippi, in exchange for room and board, but he had to leave because of inappropriate advances by the man of the household.

Black people have always been in peril in some form or fashion throughout the history of this country. We have to be careful to avoid offending those that may have some level of authority over us because they may bring distress or harm to us or our families. It is a balancing act that causes constant stress in our lives.

Like many other Black people during the Great Migration, my father was ambitious and adventurous enough to move his family out of that environment, first to Detroit in the late 1930s and then to California in the early 1950s. He worked two or three jobs to provide for us, and he became self-educated, as he read every newspaper he could get his hands on. In California, my father also possessed a top secret clearance as a truck driver delivering classified materials to the US government.

My mother enjoyed being a homemaker, cooking and caring for her family, but I was fortunate to grow up at a time when opportunities were starting to open up for women and minorities. I thought that my life could be different. If I studied hard, I could have a career and avoid some homemaker duties. Even as a young girl, I would tell my family, "I'm going to be a businesswoman and pay people to cook and clean for me."

Now, in spite of many obstacles, I had prevailed in completing my education. I had put myself through college after a disastrous marriage, while working, raising my son, and helping Thomas raise his daughter. We had both overcome so much, and we had done it together.

* * *

Graduation brought to the forefront an important change that Thomas felt he needed to make in his life—he had to file for a divorce to terminate his marriage. He had achieved a very important milestone in his life, and he felt he no longer wanted to be stuck in his past.

Even though his wife lived in Louisiana, Thomas filed for divorce in the state of California around 1977. That is where they were married, that is where he lived, and that is where his daughter, Nichelle, was living, since she was staying with us at the time. Thomas's wife never showed up to court, and he was granted a default divorce and was awarded full custody of Nichelle. However, approximately ten months later, he received a call from his attorney.

"You haven't gotten married again, have you?" he asked.

"No. Why? What's this all about?"

A California judge had thrown out the divorce and child custody decision after Thomas's wife acquired a new attorney who said that since a child was involved, the wife was not properly represented. It seemed that she believed or was advised that if she did not show up in the California court, the proceeding could not take place without her.

So now, Thomas was still legally married and aggravated about this turn of events. He and his wife ended up back in court, where the divorce was again granted in early 1979. Thomas was then awarded joint custody of his daughter with his ex-wife.

* * *

It was after Thomas's second divorce that the discussion of marriage finally came up.

"I'm surprised you're not hounding me about getting married," he said. This was Thomas's way of feeling me out without asking me directly. I had been honest with him during that first time we went out together, when I told him that I never wanted to get married again, and I still felt the same way.

"Why do I want to get married?" I asked. "I've had that piece of paper before. What did it do for me? It doesn't make anybody love me. It didn't make anyone appreciate me. It didn't make me feel safe. I don't need a piece of paper. I want a relationship. I have that now, and I'm very happy with the way things are."

Thomas listened and said nothing. He never brought up the subject again.

Then, after all that, I ended up being the one to raise the issue.

In November of 1979, I was looking over our taxes to determine ways to minimize our tax liability for that year. By then we had moved just outside Seattle, buying a home in Kirkland, Washington. The drug and gang infestation situation in Los Angeles at the time was intolerable, and I wanted to shelter our kids from that as much as possible. Examining our finances and considering that the lack of an official marriage document could have prevented us from taking care of one another, or our children, in an emergency, it made sense to get married.

"Baby," I said. "Uncle Sam is going to kill us. I have all these taxable wages with hardly any expenses. With your business, you have tons of expenses. We need to get married so we can file a joint return and pay less taxes."

Thomas did not hesitate. "Okay, Baby," he said, grinning. "Let's get married."

When deciding on a date, I thought New Year's Eve would be fun. I made an appointment at the Bellevue, Washington, courthouse for December 31, 1979 at 6:00 p.m. for our marriage ceremony.

At about 4:00 p.m. that day, Thomas was putting on his tie when he asked, "Should we do this?"

I was so focused on the tax and legal implications to getting married that it never occurred to me that Thomas might be reconsidering marriage.

"Well, if we don't do it today, then there's no rush because we'll miss the tax benefit."

Thomas said nothing. He just continued to get ready, and so did I.

When we arrived at the courthouse, we were informed that the judge presiding over the ceremony would be one Honorable Melvin Love. I gasped when I heard the name.

"Baby," I said, excitedly. "Did you know the physician that delivered me at home in Detroit was Dr. Will Thomas Love? He eventually became the first African American Medical Examiner in Wayne County, Michigan. This is amazing. Baby, I have so much love going on in my life. Love brought me into this world, our love brought us together, and now Love is going to marry us."

Thomas smiled and squeezed my hand.

And so, on December 31 at 6:00 p.m., standing in the presence of Michael, Nichelle, and our neighbors John, Diana, and their daughter Heather, with Judge Melvin Love presiding, I became Mrs. Thomas James Brown—and the world would celebrate our anniversary every year thereafter.

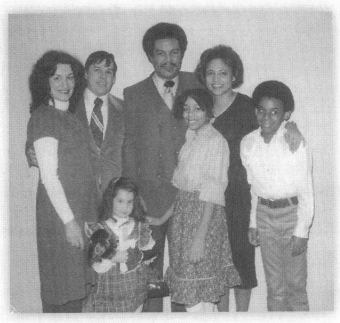

Our wedding, December 31, 1979. Bellevue, WA.
Back row: Diana & John Dolin, Thomas, Jonnie, Michael
Front row: Heather Dolin, Nichelle

* * *

When Diana and John invited us to their home afterward to present us with a card, a bottle of champagne, and a pair of champagne glasses, Thomas's uncertainty about marriage showed itself again. "You're not going to change up on me now, are you?"

I knew what he really meant. Despite our love for each other, I think he worried about a second marriage failing—that once we were married, certain aspects of our relationship would change or even go away.

"Nothing is going to change, Baby," I said. "What you have seen—and you have seen it all—will not change. No surprises."

And that was true. By the time we got married, Thomas and I had already been through so much and truly understood how we related to one another. Our love and understanding only continued to grow throughout the years.

One of the secrets to our good marriage was being friends first. We truly liked each other and had the utmost respect for one another, never calling the other anything worse than our given names. We also both guarded and protected our relationship—something that Thomas showed me how to do through his own actions—vowing to let nothing and no one come between us.

It was the small gestures of thoughtfulness that were the most meaningful to both of us, though, like always kissing one another before bed and saying, "Good morning," "Thank you," "I'm sorry," and "I love you." We enjoyed each other's company and were very content to do absolutely nothing as long as we were close to each other in the same room, especially in our later years together. We just never wanted to be separated from each other for any length of time.

* * *

John and Diana were the most wonderful, thoughtful neighbors Thomas and I had ever known, and we all became very close friends over the years. Our families spent many days together, sharing dinners and enjoying each other's company, especially in the wintertime in front of their fireplace stove in their family room.

John was employed at an aircraft manufacturer, but he was also accomplished at home repair and remodeling, often helping Thomas with various projects around the house. Diana was a homemaker and the best friend that we could ever ask for, and she demonstrated that in countless ways. Heather, their daughter, would often come across the street to visit Thomas because he would give her cookies. On one occasion, she stubbed her toe crossing the street, and Thomas cleaned and bandaged her toe for her.

Heather loved and admired Thomas very much, so it was easy to understand that when it was her turn to bring someone to "Special Person's Day" at school, Heather chose Thomas without hesitation. Heather and John headed across the street so Heather could ask Thomas to be her Special Person at school. Thomas was deeply moved by the invitation as he listened to Heather talk about the visit, when it was, and what he was supposed to do.

Thomas showed up at Heather's school at the appointed time and waited in the lobby for Heather to take him to her classroom. Off they went, a little white girl leading a six foot one—plus six inches of Afro—Black man down the hall to her kindergarten classroom. Shortly after that, Diana received a phone call from the school because they were concerned that Heather was with a Black man at school. Diana responded, "It's okay. That's just Thomas, Heather's Special Person." However, Diana and John were troubled by the phone call and at a loss for what to do next, wondering what other parents thought. It appears that Thomas's presence was perceived as threatening, requiring confirmation from someone else that he was of good character. Heather, on the other hand, was as happy as a little girl could be because Thomas was a hit with all her classmates.

John did not tell me this story until about three years after Thomas's death. He did not want me and Thomas to be offended and hurt at the time, so he kept this quiet for over forty years. As John said most recently, "Their loss, our gain because Thomas was a gentle giant and good friend."

* * *

As best friends, Thomas and I did everything together. Thomas never liked the idea of my leaving him, even when I had to travel to visit my elderly parents or for my job. Truth be told, I never liked leaving him either. In fact, I recall how my book club wanted to take a trip to a city that was the location of the book we were reading, and I told them that I could not—that I would not—go without my husband.

"Oh, girl," one of them said, "I can't wait to get away from my husband."

I never understood that feeling—the need to get away. My husband wanted me by his side, and I wanted the same. I told them I couldn't go, and I didn't.

However, despite our deep affection for each other, one situation tested our love and friendship like no other—our children. They were the only source of major disagreements between us.

Parenting is already a challenge, especially when children reach their teenage years, and it becomes more nuanced in a blended family situation. Add to that two parents who have different approaches to raising kids—combined with the special relationship that can exist between a mother and her son and a father and his daughter—and it can be even more difficult. I will be the first to admit that Thomas and I were not the best equipped to deal with all of this as we struggled to raise our kids.

Even societal factors impacted our family. I often felt that, as a stepmother, I had accepted all the responsibilities of being a mother but did not have the respect. I wanted us to be a family like any other family, but there seemed to be factors that sometimes worked against us, including family and friends.

While I cannot recall the specifics of the situation, something once happened regarding our children that caused a blow up between me and Thomas. I cursed and got so angry that I said I needed to go my own way, that I did not need this in my life, and that I did not have to put up with it. Thomas was angry too—I had never seen him so upset. His hazel eyes looked to bug right out of his head. This scared me, and I backed away from him.

Thomas realized he was scaring me, and because he could not bear to see me fearful of him, he completely changed. His tone, his facial expression, his posture—everything shifted. He sat me down on the sofa and said, "My mother told me that my wife is always number one in my life. *You* are my wife, and *you* are number one. We're *not* going to break up over our kids. In a few years, they'll be off to college, doing their own thing. We don't want to be out there trying to find someone else over this nonsense.

"You're always so quick to say you're leaving. Stop that. Don't say that anymore. We're going to be together for a long time. That's what I want, and I think you do too. Please promise me that you'll never again threaten to walk away. Promise me that next time, you won't go there. Instead, let's promise that we will focus all of our energy into resolving the problem. Promise me that we'll talk about things when they begin to bother you, instead of waiting until you are ready to blow up like this. Let's be open and honest about everything so that we both always know at any time where the other one stands."

I promised him from that day forward that we would figure out how to work on our issues without me saying I would jump ship. I really began to see the value in opening up to Thomas about things that were bothering me, without fear that he would hold it against me or that it may become grounds for us to break up—because that was not an option.

It was so comforting to know that I never had to wonder whether or not my husband and I were going to make it. Those feelings of safety and security that he gave me were more precious to me than anything else during my life with Thomas.

CHAPTER 4

LOOK HOW FAR OUR FAMILY HAS COME

AFTER THOMAS AND I GRADUATED, I CHOSE TO NOT RETURN TO the FAA because of the excitement I felt at achieving my long-held dream of a college education. I could now work in my field of study. Soon, I received several job offers from international accounting firms.

When I started my new position, however, I often felt uncomfortable around my white male colleagues, so I began regularly meeting with a group of Black accountants. All of us were members of the National Association of Black Accountants, and we gave one another the professional support we all needed in this industry that was just beginning to hire minorities.

At this time, in the mid-1970s in Los Angeles, we had an expressly stated rule among us Black accountants that we should never pose serious work questions to anyone except our fellow Black accountants. We believed that our questions only served to indicate to our bosses what we did not know, and we did not trust how we may be judged.

Therefore, we never revealed on the job what we did not understand, and we promised to be available to each other at any time for help.

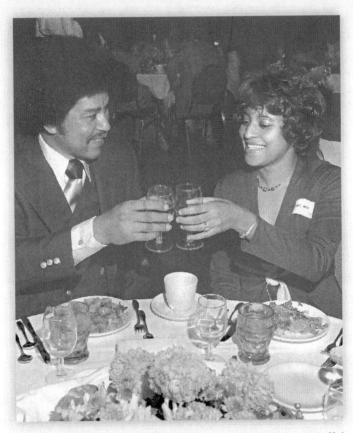

Thomas & Jonnie at Deloitte's (formerly Haskins & Sells) staff banquet. Los Angeles, CA. About 1975

During my two and a half years at a CPA (Certified Public Accountant) firm, I was required to manage an audit to complete my certification. Though I had only supported audits before, by testing transactions and developing working papers, I was assigned as audit manager of a tiny real estate company. I did not know how to begin.

So, panicked, I called my good buddy Joseph, who told me to make myself look busy until he got off work. I shuffled papers all day long until about 4:00 p.m., when Joseph arrived to point me in the right direction. My audit passed scrutiny, and I became a California CPA in December 1976.

This is how Black people were successful when we began to enter corporate America in numbers. We could not always trust others to be concerned about our general welfare, so we protected and guided each other. We would say, "Don't ever let their lack of interest or questionable behavior discourage you and make you give up. Fight back by being the best you can be. Whatever they're asking of you, learn it better than anybody else. That's how you defeat them: you do not let them defeat you."

When I decided to leave that accounting firm after two and a half years, one of the managing partners voiced that he did not want me to go. I told him that I did not think I was suited for that type of work, so he said that I had great potential and even offered to appoint someone to formally mentor me. I knew that he was trying to keep me because at that time, companies had to employ women and minorities in order to be awarded government contracts—so I just told him that I had been offered a better position.

What I did not say was that I was really leaving because I was uncomfortable. Colleagues would see me and turn their back to avoid saying hello or ignore me when I greeted them. They would act like I was not in the room or not invite me out to lunch with the group. They assumed I was less smart, and I had to work twice as hard because the bar was set higher for me—and people like me. I was confidentially told that clients did not want a woman performing audit work at their organizations, especially a Black woman.

No wonder my colleagues and I turned to the National Association of Black Accountants. It would not do any good to complain about the way we were treated; those who complained did not fare well in these organizations and were sometimes seen as troublemakers. We Black accountants knew that the best strategy, in most cases, was to gain excellent skills, move on, make more money, and always maintain a network that would lift us up.

I learned those lessons well. When I left the organization, I was now a CPA and accepted a 50 percent raise in salary on my new job. My CPA credential, along with the skills and knowledge I acquired while working for one of the largest international accounting firms, have been my golden ticket to a good job and promotion anytime I chose to move on during my career.

When Thomas and I started our careers, we decided that we wanted balanced lives. We wanted to do well at our jobs and make good money, but we also wanted to enjoy life by traveling, creating new life experiences, and supporting our kids.

Thomas worked in residential and commercial sales or as a real estate appraiser for most of his life, while I was an accountant in a variety of industries, but those jobs did not define us. When we were presented with an exciting opportunity, we were not afraid to move on. We lived in California, Washington State, Georgia, and Washington, DC, and we knew that our credentials would allow us to get jobs or start up businesses wherever we might find ourselves. We just wanted to savor life, and we worked hard so that we could do the things we enjoyed.

Like going to the Olympics.

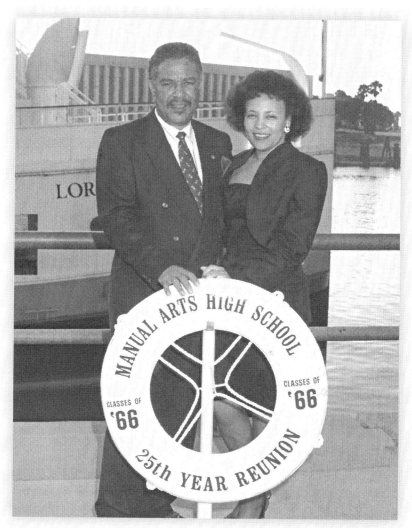

Thomas & Jonnie at Jonnie's 25th high school reunion.
Long Beach, CA. 1991

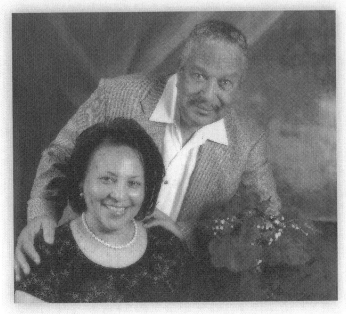

Jonnie & Thomas on a Caribbean cruise. December 2008

* * *

My son Michael was always a very rambunctious little boy. He seldom sat still, and he had difficulty quieting down when it was time to go to bed. I would often get in bed with him to rub his back so that he would relax and go to sleep.

He was constantly on the move, running and jumping. His kindergarten, first, and second grade teachers always noted that Michael would complete his classwork because it was easy for him, but then he could not sit still long enough to allow other students to finish their work. When he sat down to do homework, he would bounce one leg or the other and constantly tap his pencil on the table.

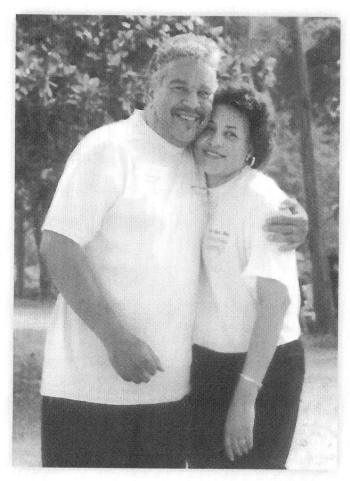

Thomas & Jonnie at the Horne, Halsell Holsey
family reunion. Detroit, MI. July 1991

My girlfriends told me I needed to take him to the doctor, that he appeared hyperactive. "Maybe he needs medication," they said. I did not pay them any mind until Michael hurt himself running around the house. He tripped and fell, cutting his mouth on a small toy car he held in his hand, and he needed stitches to close the gash.

Later, when I asked Michael's physician about the need for medications, he said, "Whoa, Mother," and ran a number of tests. When the results came back, he told me, "Mother, Michael doesn't need medication. Michael needs discipline."

There was nothing wrong with Michael medically, but he was incredibly energetic. The doctor highly recommended enrolling him in sports, telling me that if I did not do something with all that energy, Michael would, and the doctor guaranteed that I would not like what Michael came up with.

That was all I needed to hear.

I enrolled Michael in a variety of different sports programs from the time he was about four years old. Michael snow skied, played softball, bowled, and took karate classes while also participating in other activities like learning to play the clarinet. In Kirkland, Washington, around 1979, our neighbor Jim approached me to tell me that he was starting a summer track program at the park and wanted to know if Michael would be interested. I was always on the lookout for new activities for Michael to keep him busy and out of trouble, so I said yes on his behalf. Luckily, Michael was interested.

Michael continued to run track in junior high school and then throughout high school in the mid-1980s, receiving several athletic scholarship offers from such universities as Brown, Cornell, University of Washington, and more. Of course, I was elated at these developments, since track had started out as a means for him to burn off all that excess energy and stay out of trouble. On the occasions where Michael would act up or act out, I never punished him by taking away his participation in track activities because I saw them as a medical prescription from the doctor. Besides, Michael truly loved the sport, and I marveled at how focused he was at trying to excel at his events.

When he was in high school, Michael's track activities took us to many states in the country. I was fortunate enough to never miss a trip because I had great jobs that offered flexibility and great bosses who understood my need to support my son. Thomas joined us whenever he could get away from his business.

While Michael was attending UCLA, and afterward, Thomas and I traveled overseas many times to his track events. Track-and-field is a major sport in Europe, comparable to football and basketball in the United States. We had so much fun at track meets on the European track circuit in Germany, Sweden, Italy, France, Monaco, and other countries, as the crowd was boisterous and rowdy, but they policed themselves and quieted down when the athletes were at the starting line for the beginning of a race. Michael was a celebrity in these over-seas locations, which made me and Thomas celebrities in our own right once people found out we were his parents.

But never did I imagine we were raising an Olympian.

Can you imagine? Michael's success in track took him to the 1988 Olympics in Seoul, Korea, the 1992 Olympics in Barcelona, Spain, and the 1996 Olympics in Atlanta, Georgia. In Barcelona, he gold medaled—twice—and set American and Olympic records in the 200-meter dash and a world record as the lead-off man on the 4x100 meter relay. In Atlanta, he earned a silver medal in the 4x100 meter relay.

In 1988, prior to the Seoul Olympics, I told Thomas that if my boss did not allow me to take two weeks off to attend, I was prepared to quit my job. This was a once-in-a-lifetime opportunity, and no job would keep me from supporting Michael and experiencing something that few parents can ever imagine. Thomas agreed. When I presented my plan to my boss, Al, demonstrating how my work would get done on time in my absence, Al said, "Of course you have to go. Have fun and enjoy every minute of it."

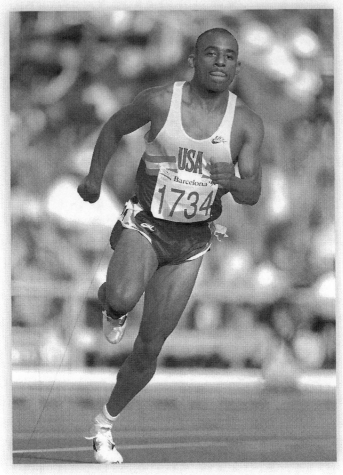

My son, Michael. 200-meter gold medalist.
1992 Olympic Games in Barcelona, Spain.

I remember vividly in 1992 when Michael let me bring the two gold medals home that he won in Barcelona so I could show them off to all my friends and coworkers. When Thomas and I went through security at JFK Airport, they set off the alarm. The guard wanted to know if, in fact, they were real Olympic medals. When I said, "Yes, they belong to my son, Michael Marsh," he called over some of his coworkers to see.

The next thing I knew, they were treating Thomas and me like VIPs, like *we* had won the medals. They offered us drink coupons and asked if there were any changes we wanted to make to our flight. I asked Thomas if we could reroute our flight through Atlanta, since Atlanta would be hosting the next Olympics in 1996. Our entire family, including Michael and Nichelle as teenagers, had worked for the 1984 Olympics in Los Angeles. Thomas was manager of the basketball venue. I thought it would be exciting to work for an Olympic organizing committee again, especially since Michael planned to try out for the USA team in 1996.

Working for an Olympic organizing committee is an exhilarating experience because the Olympics are the largest peacetime event in the world. It is a very unique opportunity to be a part of history. In fact, Michael once said that it was the roar of the crowd at the fencing venue in 1984, when he was a parking lot attendant, that made him seriously consider the possibility of becoming an Olympian.

Sure enough, the airline rerouted us and let us stay in Atlanta for four days before we flew home in first class to Seattle. We stayed with my niece Peaches, visiting with her and checking out neighborhoods where we could live. Then, on that trip back to Seattle, we decided that we were going to relocate to Atlanta so I could work for the Olympics. Thomas was not that crazy about going South, but he did not mind supporting me. We were spontaneous about many things that we did during our lives together.

We made the move to Metro Atlanta in May 1993, and I snagged my job at the Atlanta Committee for the Olympic Games shortly thereafter, working in the accounting department and later as the Business Operations Manager for the athlete Olympic Village. The latter was a dream job. During the Games, I managed the National Olympic Committee (NOC) Center, where we fielded every question imaginable from the administrative heads from all of the 197 participating countries.

Michael retired from track in 2000, after an injury hampered his performance at the Olympic trials, but he was prepared for the next phase of his life, having received a full scholarship to Duke University for his MBA. I was so inspired by this accomplishment that I decided to start a fully accredited online MBA program myself through California State University, Dominguez Hills. I had observed all of these bright, young MBA graduates and realized that I needed to remain competitive.

It would take three years for me to complete my program if I paid for and enrolled in one class each quarter, but I figured three years were going to pass whether I earned a master's degree or not. So in 2004, thirty years after receiving my bachelor's degree, I graduated with Thomas by my side.

My parents were elderly then, and it was difficult for them to attend an event in a large venue. In addition, most of our friends and other family members were busy with other obligations and graduations when we notified them at the last minute that we would be coming to Los Angeles for my graduation. So Thomas and I attended my ceremony in Los Angeles alone.

I did not mind. Once again, it was the two of us showing the world that we were constantly making the best of our lives.

* * *

Like most Black men, Michael experiences a greater frequency of police contacts, discretionary stops, and police harassment when stops occur, as compared to his white counterparts. And as a parent of a Black son, I had "the talk" with him about how he should conduct himself when he has a police encounter. Keep both hands in plain sight. No sudden moves. Be respectful. Use formal English. Talk intelligently. Obey. Do not try to reason with belligerent cops; you will not prevail. Memorize the badge numbers, even the last four digits, and we will resolve all matters later under more favorable circumstances.

Michael told me that he is routinely stopped by the police. He is no longer surprised and shaken because his expectation is that he will be targeted because he is Black. As an athlete, he learned to deal with fear and panic and to think on his feet, so he is able to utilize these skills to manage his emotions and keep his body relaxed, not tense, during police stops.

One stop that was particularly disturbing occurred in Hawthorne, California, a small community just south of Los Angeles, when Michael was a freshman at UCLA. To return to the campus, Michael had made a legal left turn onto Imperial Highway heading west to Interstate 405. He was not speeding, and there was no other legitimate reason for the two white policemen to pull him over.

When Michael asked the officer why he was pulled over, the officer responded that his taillight was out. "No, Officer, I don't believe it is," Michael replied. My father had taught Michael to frequently check the head and taillights, brake lights, and the turn signals to ensure they are always in working order—to eliminate these reasons for a police stop. Michael truly believed that he would be able to show the officer that the taillight was working and then he would be on his way.

The officer told Michael to exit the vehicle, but after Michael unbuckled his seat belt, the officer yanked him out of his vehicle, bending his body over the hood. The officer held both of Michael's hands behind his back, put an elbow in his back, and leaned over and whispered in Michael's ear, "Don't ever mouth off to me again. I can kill you right now, and who do you think they are going to believe?"

The second policeman snatched Michael's wallet out of his rear pants pocket while the first policeman continued roughing Michael up. "Just show me the drugs now," the first cop said, as he made more threats about what he could do to him without repercussions. Michael felt that he was viewed and treated as someone worthless just because he was young and Black.

"Whoa, whoa, slow up," the second cop said when Michael's UCLA identification card was found in his wallet. That university ID, "a white credential," changed everything, Michael believes. The cops knew that someone was going to care about this young Black man, so the first cop released his hold on Michael—but not before asking sarcastically what his major was, still not convinced that Michael was not a criminal but a law-abiding citizen and a college student at a prestigious university like UCLA.

There is little wonder why police interactions are perceived within the Black community as harassment and disrespect. Michael's incident also explains why police legitimacy is questioned and trust in law enforcement is low.

* * *

A few years prior to moving to Atlanta, I became curious about my family history. "Daddy, where are all our relatives?" I asked my father. "I don't know any of my cousins or grandparents. Where are all of them?" We didn't travel to Mississippi when I was growing up because, as my father explained, he wanted to shelter us from the harsh realities of segregation and discrimination in Mississippi, so I didn't have the opportunity to meet my grandparents. As a result of my curiosity, my father and I began having frequent conversations about his and my mother's families.

Daddy told fascinating stories about our family. I learned that after my parents moved to Detroit, Daddy decided to apply for a job with the city bus company around the early 1940s, where his half-brother,

Walter King Johnson, already worked. My uncle was very fair, and many people did not know he was Black, so he was hired as a bus driver without issue. He told my father, "I drive my route at midnight, so just come get on the bus with me and I'll show you everything you need to know to pass the tests."

Daddy passed all of the required tests with flying colors, but during the physical, the company physician told my father that he had a terminal illness. He said that Daddy would be dead in a year, that he needed to go home and figure out how he was going to take care of his family.

Terribly upset, Daddy consulted his own doctor, who said, "You're a healthy man. There's nothing wrong with you whatsoever. They misrepresented your health to avoid hiring you. That's what this is all about." Company management and their doctor had no conscience about how this false diagnosis of impending death impacted my father and our family.

Daddy's doctor went on to tell my father that the NAACP had been looking for a case like this, and he should contact them. The NAACP filed an appeal arguing that the bus company's doctor had fabricated a disqualifying medical condition, and that my father was eligible for the bus driver position in every respect. Despite the evidence, the appeal board stood by their decision, confirming that they would not hire my father.

When my father arrived home, however, a telegram was awaiting him, stating he should report to work. It seems the company and the appeal board did not want the official record to document that the bus company doctor had intentionally lied or to document the hiring of a Black person, but because the NAACP was involved, they quietly hired him to avoid a lawsuit. That is how my father got this enviable position that raised our family's standard of living and gave my father the necessary resources to move our family to Los Angeles in the early 1950s, the land of opportunity and beautiful weather.

Many years later, once I had moved to Atlanta, my father came to visit and told me he was taking me on a field trip to Toomsuba, Mississippi, to show me the community where he was born and raised. During that trip, my interest in my family and Thomas's family deepened. I even met many cousins in Toomsuba and, on my way back home, in Birmingham.

Though I have built my repertoire of family stories over the years as a self-appointed family historian, I loved the genealogy project my grandson, Wren, completed, which was supported by documents and artifacts of four generations of our family: Wren, Michael, me, and my father. When discussing the project with Michael, I talked about how Daddy was born in a tiny, three-room, wooden house built by his father and how his quest for education was cut short but how those events did not stop him from achieving. I talked about how I was the first one in the family to achieve a college education, how he and I both have MBAs, how he has a second master's degree, how he carried the USA flag in world-class track meets around the world, and how his sons have many more opportunities than my father or I could ever imagine. It was evident how each generation had advanced beyond the last.

I said, "Look how far our family has come."

But my grandson Wren put it best in 2022 in a scholarship application for Howard University. Wren won that scholarship by writing a poignant essay about my father and the political and social events of his time. Wren concluded with: "I proudly accept the charge of carrying on the Ramsey Family tradition of upward mobility."

* * *

Over time, Thomas and I met many respective cousins online and took several trips to meet them in person. We enjoyed getting to know members of our extended family, especially Thomas, since he was able to reconnect with many cousins who did not know or care that his branch of the family were outcasts decades earlier.

My family was big on reunions, and it was not long before I found myself hosting reunions in Atlanta for both my mother's and father's side of the family. Atlanta was a city where everyone wanted to visit, so I hosted whenever it was convenient for me to do so.

In 2015, my mother turned one hundred years old. She was the last one living of her ten siblings, and I wanted our whole family to get together to celebrate her epic birthday. Sadly, she died before that could come to pass, but I had committed to the reunion and decided to hold it in her honor regardless.

The 2017 family reunion was on the verge of being canceled, so I offered to host again. Reunions were relatively easy for me to plan and execute because of my special events experience at two Olympic organizing committees. Only eight months remained to plan the 2017 reunion, but I felt confident I could make it happen.

It is a decision I will regret for the rest of my life.

CHAPTER 5

I TOLD YOU
WHAT THE PLAN WAS

MOST EVERYONE IN THE FAMILY DID *NOT* WANT TO COME TO Atlanta again for the 2017 reunion, so I researched several cities— Charleston, Savannah, New Orleans, Memphis, etc. I eventually settled on Greater Orlando because planning various events would be relatively easy since there were so many activities that people could do on their own.

Because of my love for genealogy and our family history, I decided to create a book of family stories as a gift for the attendees. I asked cousins to write stories and locate photographs of their parents and grandparents, and I planned to combine those with official documents I had discovered in my research. I was going to highlight the first three generations coming out of slavery on my mother's side of the family. My mother was the last of the third generation, and I did not want all of that history that my older cousins and I possessed to be lost should something happen to us.

So, I was working on the book, planning for the reunion, and working my full-time job. Between those three things, I often found myself going to bed at five or six in the morning, then remotely logging onto my job at 9:00 a.m. Except for sleeping in on Saturdays and Sundays, I was not getting much rest at all.

In the meantime, despite his love of cooking, Thomas had gotten to a point where he didn't want to cook as much but wanted to be served. We went out to eat often—but that was time consuming.

"Baby, I can't go out for two hours a night, three times a week," I said. "That's six hours every week where I could be working on all the things I've got to do. You go ahead and eat and bring me back something. I *promise* you, once we get back from the family reunion, we can do whatever you want."

Thomas hated eating by himself, but he did anyway, and he always brought something home for me.

If I could take every one of those hours back, I would. The thought of him sitting alone in the restaurant pains me so much. Given the chance to do it all over again, I would have been by his side every time he asked me to dinner.

I had no way of knowing those several months leading up to the reunion would be the last months of his life.

* * *

I managed to get everything done for the reunion on time. The books were delivered to our home three days prior to our departure, and we rented an SUV for the trip. My SUV was older, so we did not trust putting it on the road for the seven-hour drive to Orlando, and Thomas's truck was not appropriate because I did not want to put anything in the bed of the truck in case of rain.

The weekend before Wednesday, July 19, when we had planned to leave for Orlando, Thomas started feeling like he had a cold. The day before we left, however, he said he was better.

Then on Wednesday, July 19, when loading the car, Thomas told me, "Baby, I don't feel well."

"Well, I'm not ready, anyway," I said. "In fact, I'm nowhere near ready. I haven't even packed yet. Don't rush and push yourself. Go ahead and sit down and relax whenever you feel you need to do so."

I did not really pay him any mind. Thomas was a diabetic and a cancer survivor, and though both of us took his health seriously, I was normally the one pushing him to go to the doctor at the slightest hint that something was wrong. But in my rush to get ready, I just did not think that this was anything to worry about.

By the time I had finished everything I needed to do, it was around 7:00 p.m.—and Thomas, well, he was upset, and rightfully so. He did not want to drive such a long distance in the dark, especially when he was not feeling well. I had told him we would leave by noon so we could maximize our time driving in daylight, but I had not actually gotten out of bed until close to 12:00 p.m. that day. I had been so tired, putting in so many hours to prepare, that I just could not wake up any earlier.

"There's nothing we can do now," I said. "We have to leave tonight. The reunion starts tomorrow. Let's just do whatever it takes. If we have to stop every hour, then we'll stop every hour."

I volunteered to take the first shift driving, but after about an hour, I could not drive anymore. I was so tired, and the white lines on the highway were hypnotizing. Thomas, bless him, said he would drive the rest of the way, despite his not feeling nor looking well.

I fell asleep in the passenger seat but woke often to check on him. When I pressed him to tell me exactly what he was feeling, he described common cold symptoms, but nothing more severe than that.

"Do you feel okay?" I asked. "Do you want me to drive? I can."

Thomas said no. He knew that I had difficulties driving at night.

* * *

There was another time, approximately three years prior, when Thomas had complained of severe cold symptoms. He had reacted in the same way then, saying he was fine and that he would simply ride it out. He cannot take over-the-counter medications due to his diabetes, so he said he would simply let the bug run its course.

However, the symptoms landed him in bed for a few days. When he measured his blood sugar, it was always on the high side, around 160 mg/dL or so (less than 140 mg/dL is considered normal). As a result, he ate as little as possible, mainly drinking diabetic shakes, hoping his sugar would drop.

When Thomas finally felt better, he went to the doctor. His primary care doctor told him in no uncertain terms to never do that again—the next time he was sick like that, he was to come see him immediately.

Thomas loved his primary care doctor at Everett Clinic in Atlanta. He was an excellent communicator, and Thomas appreciated doctors who took the time to explain things rather than making the patient figure out the right questions to ask.

I recalled when Thomas was diagnosed with prostate cancer in 2011. I was working for the Department of Homeland Security in Washington, DC, at the time, and Thomas had retired. Though we rented a small apartment in Maryland, we kept our house in the Atlanta area and continued receiving our healthcare at Everett. We would come home every two or three months to take care of business, to check on my elderly mother who now resided in Atlanta, and to see our doctors.

I had attended all of Thomas's early cancer appointments with him when the doctors were discussing the potential treatment methods available to him. I was the one who asked what Thomas's likelihood for survival was.

"Oh, he's going to make it," the urologist said.

"What makes you so sure?"

"I've done this for a long time. I know the ones I can cure, and seeing the stage Mr. Brown is in, I know he's going to be fine."

Even with the doctor's assurances, I was nervous. Meanwhile, Thomas seemed to go about his days as usual, not saying much, if anything at all, about the diagnosis. A few days after that appointment, I needed to know his state of mind.

"Baby, tell me how you feel. Tell me what you're thinking."

He paused for a moment. Then he looked directly at me. "Never for one moment did I think I wasn't going to make it, Baby."

Well, alrighty then, I remember thinking. I was so glad to hear that Thomas was that positive about his cancer recovery. He believed that he would survive, and so I did too.

* * *

My first thought upon hearing of Thomas's cancer diagnosis was that we needed to find medical facilities in the DC area for Thomas's cancer treatment, but Thomas was adamant.

"No, Baby. Everett diagnosed this cancer, I'm in the queue for tests and consultations, and I don't want to try to establish a new relationship with another hospital that I've never been to before."

"But, Baby," I said. "What am I going to do? I have to work in DC. I can't leave you here by yourself to deal with this alone."

"I'll be fine, Baby. You go back to work and come back as often as you can because I'm getting my care at Everett."

I was not back in DC for one week before Thomas called me and said, "Baby, I need you here with me."

"Okay, Baby. Oh my goodness. Let me see what arrangements I can work out with my boss, and we'll talk later tonight."

I remember it was December 7, 2011. I studied my work calendar so that I could come up with a workable schedule that allowed me to spend as much time as possible at home in the next six and a half weeks, the length of time for Thomas's radiation treatments. My proposed work schedule called for two weeks of vacation at the end of December, returning to DC for a week and a half in January for our busy quarter-end activities, and then I would use a combination of other vacation days, telework days, and holidays to make up the rest of the time.

I presented my request to my boss, Melissa, and she rose from her chair and went to the calendar on the wall. "So, Jonnie, you want vacation at the end of the month, then you'll be in the office, then telework...just forget all this, Jonnie. Go home and take care of your husband. I know you'll do whatever you need to do to get your work done, so go telework at home and take care of Thomas."

I was overcome, hearing Melissa say all this. I was so grateful to her for understanding how important it was for me to care for my husband at that difficult time.

* * *

On the drive to Orlando, we stopped and got coffee and food a few times so that Thomas could stay awake, and all the way he declined my offers to take over driving. I asked over and over again, but he insisted that I was the one who was tired—that I was one who needed the rest.

After almost seven hours on the road, we arrived in Orlando early Thursday morning, July 20, about 2:30 a.m. We unloaded the car and got everything up to the hotel room. Thomas fell into bed when we were done and was asleep within minutes.

Later that morning, Thomas awoke for breakfast as he usually did, careful to eat on time as part of his diabetes regimen. He was always good about staying on track with his meals and keeping his blood sugar under control.

After we had a quick bite in the dining area, we saw some of my cousins who had already arrived. Thomas and I joined them at one of the tables. Everyone was smiling and laughing and greeting one another, catching up on happenings in their lives. I left the table to mingle, leaving Thomas to talk with my cousin Larry.

Two or three weeks later, Larry would tell me that when they sat together, the conversation took a dark turn. Thomas said to Larry that if anything ever happened to him—if he were to get severely ill—that he did not want to lay in bed, wasting away. His grandfather had been bedridden for more than seven years and he could not imagine going out like that, unable to even wipe his own backside. Larry told me he did not know why the conversation went in that direction, but he remembered that Thomas seemed fixated on the idea.

It reminded me of a conversation I had with Thomas the year prior.

Thomas was in the kitchen cooking when he said, "Baby, what would you do if anything ever happened to me?" He knew that I essentially depended on him for everything. He took such good care of me.

"Oh, nothing's going to happen to you," I said, smiling. "I want to be a centenarian. I'm going to live to be 100. That means you need to live to be 106. After that, we can both go together."

"Wow, Baby. But I'm not going to make it to 106, so you have to come up with another plan."

We both laughed then. But just months before the trip to Orlando, he brought it up in a different way—in a way where things were not so funny—more of a statement rather than a question. We were together in the kitchen again.

"Baby, I don't know what you're going to do without me if something ever happened."

"Baby, I told you what the plan was." I tried to laugh it off, but Thomas was not joining in this time. But this was not a subject I wanted to think about, so I did not.

* * *

I spent most of the rest of the first day of the reunion greeting family and coordinating with the hotel to make sure everything was set up just right for the meet and greet that evening. Meanwhile, Thomas returned to our room to get some more rest. Time flew by, and when I finally came up, it was time for us to get ready for the evening's event.

Back downstairs, Thomas sat at a table by himself. He did not say a word to anyone, which was so unlike him. Once again, he did not look well, so I went over to him to see if he was okay. He told me not to worry about him and to "go be the gracious hostess."

"Do you want me to get you a plate of food? They put out quite a spread." I knew he didn't like anyone fixing his plate—Thomas was meticulous about the presentation of his food on his plate—but I asked anyway because he looked so tired.

"No, no," he said. "I'll get me something."

He got up and fixed himself a plate while I continued to float from family member to family member. I stole more glances at Thomas alone at the table. From time to time, people would come up and say hello to him, but he did not say much, other than returning the greeting. When I found another spare moment, I returned to him at the table.

"You look terrible, Baby."

Thomas smiled weakly. "I feel terrible," he said. "I think I'm going back up to the room. I can't stay down here anymore."

"Baby, do you want me to walk you back to the room?" I asked, worried. "Or I can get someone to walk you back if you want."

"No, no, no, I'm fine. But I'm going back. I just want to lay down, Baby."

I did not want to argue with him. Thomas got up from the table and went upstairs to bed. Eventually, the festivities wound down, and I returned to the room, exhausted. Thomas awoke briefly, but by the time I climbed into bed, he had already fallen asleep again. I went to sleep soon after—concerned, but with no idea what was about to come.

CHAPTER 6

WHY DON'T YOU GET OUT OF BED?

For Friday morning, July 21, I had planned a breakfast meeting at 10:00 a.m. with the family. My plans for that meeting consisted of a formal welcome, introductions, writing letters to our family that would be placed in a "time capsule" to be opened years from then, a gifting game, and presentation of our family history book. That afternoon at 2:00 p.m., lunch was scheduled at the House of Blues at Disney Springs. Everyone would then have free time for the rest of the evening where they could hang out wherever they wanted to—at Disney Springs, the entertainment areas close to the hotel, or anywhere else they chose.

I was excited about the gifting game, where people could take each other's gifts during the course of the game, if they preferred that gift over theirs. I had brought gifts for everyone—photo albums, mugs with clever sayings, beach towels, wall hangings with family sayings on them, lottery tickets, fancy luggage tags, pistachio nuts, and bags of candy for the kids. This was a relatively small reunion with about fifty family members in attendance, but nevertheless, there was a lot to do to prepare for that morning meeting.

In order to have everything ready, I woke up early. Thomas woke up as well, and I asked him for his help to put the gift bags together.

"Ask someone else to help you," he said.

"Some of these are surprises," I told him. "I don't want anybody else to see what they might win."

"Well, I don't feel like it."

"All you have to do is sit there on the couch and I'll give you the gift, the bag, and the tissue paper. You don't even have to move."

He begrudgingly agreed. Once we finished, I looked around the room and realized that of the three boxes of books I had asked Thomas to pack in the car, there were only two. When I asked him where the third was, he insisted I had only set out two for the trip.

The books were a gift for anyone who attended the reunion, but I needed extras for anyone who wanted to purchase additional copies. I overreacted when Thomas told me he had not brought the third box.

"You ruined everything," I said.

Thomas did not say anything. When I realized how I had overreacted, I apologized, telling him, "Baby, I'm sorry. I'm just tired." I told him that if anyone wanted to buy books, I could simply mail them later.

He accepted my apology by responding with one simple word. "Yes."

Oh, how I look back on that moment with such regret.

When it came time to go down for the family meeting at 10:00 a.m., I asked Thomas to come downstairs with me, but he continued to say he did not feel well.

"No," he said. "I'm just going to lay here in bed. I still don't feel good."

"Okay, well make sure you get up and go eat some breakfast at some point." I put two bottles of water on the nightstand. "Make sure you get some fluids in you. Drink these, okay, Baby?"

I was hoping Thomas would join us for lunch at the House of Blues that afternoon, but he did not. I rushed back to the room after lunch to check on him.

He was still in bed. He had not drunk any of his water. He had not gone down to the hotel restaurant to get breakfast or lunch.

"Why don't you get out of bed?" I asked.

No matter how often I asked him to get out of bed and get himself something to eat, he refused. He just wanted to lay in bed.

And that is where he stayed for the rest of the day.

* * *

The next morning, Saturday, July 22, we had a quilting activity planned for the family. My cousin Shirley first introduced me to quilting and taught me about its importance in African American history, so I was particularly excited to partake in this event with the family. After the quilting activity, everyone would be on their own for lunch, and then that evening we would all get dressed up for a fancy sit-down dinner.

I woke up early again so I could help Shirley with the setup for her presentation. Thomas told me he still was not feeling well. He got up to use the bathroom, closing the door behind him. I continued to rush around the room, figuring out what I was going to wear that morning.

When he finally came out, I dashed into the bathroom to take a shower—only to find that Thomas had urinated all over the floor.

It was not a near miss. It was not on the seat. There was a large puddle on the floor.

Thomas seemed not to have noticed. He plopped down on the couch while I stood in the bathroom, dumbstruck.

"Baby, you peed on the floor!"

At that, there was a knock on the door. The hotel maid wanted to come in to do her rounds. I told her that my husband was not feeling well and had urinated all over the bathroom floor. I asked her if she would clean it up, as well as change out our bed linens. She agreed, and I told her I was ever so grateful before I turned my attention back to Thomas back on the couch.

"Baby, we have to get you to the doctor."

"No," he said. "I don't want to go to the doctor."

"Thomas, you have to go. This has never happened to you before."

Still, he refused.

"You promised me. Remember that you promised me that the next time that I made the call that you needed to go to the doctor that you weren't going to argue with me. I'm making the call. You've had these cold symptoms going back to last weekend. Now you're peeing on the floor like you're delirious or something. Something is wrong, Baby. You're going, Baby."

Thomas knew the promise he had made to me about agreeing to see the doctor when I said so, and we always honored our promises to one another. "Okay," he said.

"Okay." I got a washcloth to clean him up, as well as some clean clothes, and helped him get dressed. My cousin Tommy came to our room to pray for Thomas before we headed out to see the doctor.

"Do you want to hold on to me?" I asked Thomas as we walked out of the room.

"No, I'm fine."

"Well, *I'm* holding on," I said.

Thomas wanted me to believe he was strong, but I could feel him leaning his weight into me. I could not imagine how he had gotten so weak. We made it to the elevator, down to the lobby, and up to the front desk, where I asked about an urgent care close to the hotel that could be recommended. The desk clerk provided me with the addresses to several, and I drove to the closest one.

Once there, I filled out all the necessary paperwork while Thomas rested in a chair. Eventually, Thomas's name was called, and I accompanied him into the exam room. The doctor performed the typical cursory examination, listening with his stethoscope and looking into Thomas's eyes, ears, nose, and throat.

"I don't think I can treat him here," he finally said. "I really think he needs to go to a hospital for blood work. He's dehydrated, and we don't do IV fluids here. There's a brand-new Veterans Medical Center close to here. There is also Viewpark Hospital, which isn't too far from the hotel where you say your reunion is being held."

The VA hospitals had been experiencing controversy for many years about the quality of their healthcare, and Thomas had told me on several occasions to *never* take him to a VA hospital under any circumstances.

"We have insurance," Thomas said. "Don't take me to the VA."

I agreed, and we decided to go to Viewpark Hospital, which was just a few miles away.

We pulled up to the emergency department there, and a Black orderly came out with a wheelchair. Thomas gave me his wallet as he climbed into the wheelchair, and I noticed the orderly wore a cap indicating he was a Vietnam veteran, similar to the one Thomas was wearing.

"Okay, soldier," he said to Thomas. "We're going to take good care of you. You don't have to worry about anything."

When he said that, I felt this overwhelming sense of relief. *He's going to be okay*, I thought. Though the hospital was small, it looked new and well funded, which also made me feel better about our decision to go there. The grounds were manicured, the admittance area was freshly painted and clean with relatively new furniture. I figured Thomas would get an IV, maybe some medications, and we would be out of there in time to get back to the hotel for the banquet.

I did not think Thomas would be up for going to the banquet, but I had to get back since no one else knew my plans for the evening. I looked at my watch and saw it was around 1:00 p.m. I calculated that we could spend four hours in the hospital and still have plenty of time for me to get ready to host the banquet that evening.

The admissions person took Thomas's insurance cards and medical information. At the time, I was still working for the federal government, so Thomas was covered under my Blue Cross Blue Shield (BCBS) health insurance. He also had Medicare, but as long as I was still working, the BCBS was the primary insurance for him. We did not have to wait long before Thomas was taken back to an examination room.

Thomas had a slight temperature, about 99.4 degrees Fahrenheit. His blood sugar was somewhat elevated, but his blood pressure was normal at 125/61. The hospital performed several additional tests. His cardiovascular rate and rhythms were regular, and his respiratory rate was in the normal range. He had generalized weakness and a low appetite. Nothing seemed immediately alarming.

Until Thomas urinated on himself again when they took him for his chest X-ray.

His lungs were clear, but Dr. Chad, the emergency physician in charge, recommended that Thomas stay overnight for observation, as he was concerned about the sudden incontinence. Thomas did *not* like hospitals, so I had to beg him to stay. I told him they would monitor him and take care of him, and then I would not have to worry about him while I was tending to the banquet that evening.

Thomas reluctantly agreed. Even while sick and in the hospital, he always supported me—always put me first to alleviate my worries.

I promised to return after the banquet, no matter the time, and then I rushed back to the hotel. Once there, I called on several cousins to come up to my room with a cart to bring all of the items I needed for the banquet. After they had left, I had just enough time to shower and get dressed.

I made it downstairs just a few minutes after the scheduled start time. The word had already gotten around about Thomas being admitted to the hospital, so everyone was patient about my being late, asking only about how he and I were doing.

My family was not the only one waiting for me—the hotel sales manager was there too. She informed me that I owed the hotel approximately $1,500 for not meeting the contracted number of booked rooms. I told her I would meet with her as soon as I had the chance, most likely the next day. Thankfully, she agreed.

I then proceeded to announce to the family that Thomas was not feeling well and that he was at the hospital for observation. I told them that he would want us to enjoy ourselves, to be present in the here and now, and that is what we were going to do. I then asked everyone to gather outside of the banquet room for a group picture in front of the waterfall in the lobby. When they returned, we would have the blessing of the food and dinner would be served.

The after-dinner program showcased two of my younger cousins, Nailah on the cello and Kimi on the violin, who played three or four selections throughout the evening. My grandsons, Wren, Asa, and Maverick, spoke in honor of the servicemen in our family, distributing token gifts to all of the men. We also honored our elderly, our "Living Legacies," who all received their gifts: a collage of pictures of their closest relatives. Finally, we honored those who had passed away.

Katerri, a cousin with a spectacular singing voice, broke into a rendition of the chorus to Sean "Puffy" Combs's "I'll Be Missing You." While she was singing, family members came to the front of the room one by one, picked up a long stem rose, and placed the rose in a vase while saying the name of the family member who had died. Katerri ad-libbed some of the lyrics and added her gospel touch to the song. It was a beautiful and touching ceremony.

Catherine O'Neal, my cousin and one of the oldest family members in attendance, delivered special remarks about the family and the reunion. Zoe, my grandniece, then extended an invitation to all to attend the next family reunion in 2019. My cousin Tommy said the closing prayer.

The program ended, and the DJ played music late into the evening. The family danced and socialized, took pictures, hugged, and promised to stay in touch until the next reunion. I stayed until almost everyone left, though some hung back and helped me clean up and take supplies back to my room.

It was almost 1:00 a.m. by the time we finished, but as soon as I was able, I jumped in the car and drove as fast as I could to the hospital to see Thomas. When I arrived, he was awake in his room, waiting for me.

"I thought you weren't going to come back," he said.

I knew him well enough to know that was his way of telling me he needed me by his side.

"You knew I was coming back, Baby," I said. "I just had to tend to the family, this being the last night and all. I'm sorry I took so long."

Thomas ignored that. "I want to leave tomorrow."

"Don't worry. I'll bring you some clean clothes and hopefully you'll be released. Remember, though, we had already planned to have a relaxing day on Sunday, and then head home on Monday by noon so we can drive in the daylight. When you're released tomorrow, we'll go back to the hotel and relax for the day, okay?"

Thomas agreed. I stayed with him for another hour or so, but the day had worn me down. I was ready to head back to the hotel to get some sleep.

The next morning, Sunday, July 23, I woke up and had a small breakfast at the hotel before heading over to the hospital. I brought clean clothes, as I had promised, and was excited for Thomas's release.

But that was not to be.

Thomas's temperature had skyrocketed to 104.5. The hospital staff told me he could not be released on that day, and likely not the next day because at the moment, they did not know what was happening to him. The doctor wanted at least twenty-four hours of a normal temperature before they would release him.

In the meantime, Thomas got weaker and weaker, and he repeatedly said he was not feeling well at all. I kept thinking about how I was going to get him home. *What if he needs medical attention while we're on the road? He is so weak—how would he go to the restroom on his own? How would I handle any emergencies we might encounter? What if we were in the middle of nowhere and he needed help? Maybe we should stay at the hotel until he feels better.*

My mind raced with every imaginable scenario. All the while, I received texts and calls from family and friends checking in on Thomas. One cousin suggested that I call the Veterans Administration, as they would provide transportation to get a vet home if they were stuck out of town and needed assistance. I thanked her and kept the information in the back of my mind.

Despite the high fever, Thomas was more or less himself. We talked throughout the day. There were times when he would get sleepy and would need a nap, and I would take that time to find something to eat or a place where I could sit and think about the things I needed to do. While Thomas was sick, we were racking up a hotel bill, but all I could think about was, *How do I get him home?*

Around 7:00 p.m. on Sunday evening, I really began to get scared. Thomas's temperature simply would not go down, and even when it dropped minutely, it was only temporary. I remembered that Thomas had a urinary tract infection (UTI) earlier in the month, and I started to wonder if somehow that might have resulted in an infection that got into his bloodstream.

Just then, the hospital's Rapid Response Team came in to check on Thomas, which scared me even more. I had no idea who they were or why they were there. One of Thomas's nurses told me that they were a team that came to check on patients so that if he were to take a turn for the worse, they would be familiar with his situation and could act quickly.

When I asked them what was wrong, they responded with a phrase that would become quite common throughout our whole ordeal there: "I don't know."

* * *

Around 8:00 p.m., Thomas's temperature lowered some but then spiked again. He was conscious and alert, but even he knew this was serious.

The doctor ordered a CT scan of Thomas's lower thoracic region to see if there was another source of the infection. Approximately an hour later, at 9:00 p.m., Thomas was moved to the progressive care unit

(PCU)—a step up from the regular floor, but not quite intensive care. The team told me they moved him there because that unit was better equipped to get his temperature under control; they eventually got it down to just above 101 degrees. The nurses put ice packs under his arms and on his forehead. They gave him Tylenol and ibuprofen and watched him closely for sepsis, a serious blood infection.

Maybe because it was a way for me to quantify any improvement in his condition, I continually asked one of the PCU nurses to take his temperature. Eventually, she handed me a hand thermometer.

"Dear," she said. "Take this. You can check his temp any time you want. We're still going to come in every couple of hours to officially check it, but take this so you can check it whenever you like."

Her tone was kind. She was not trying to get rid of me, at least not that I could tell. She saw it gave me comfort to check for changes in his temperature at my discretion—and she was right.

Thomas and I continued to talk. He asked me if I had told the doctors everything about his health situation, about the medications he was on, and about the twenty-five pounds he had lost the last several months while on a weight loss and nutrition program. I told him that I had, which seemed to calm him somewhat.

Thomas napped on and off, and when he would wake, he would look around the room for me, relaxing when he saw me at his bedside. There were times when he was alert, and we could talk. There were times when he slept. There were times when he did not want to be bothered.

My worries mounted. I hated being out of town and away from Thomas's doctor, away from our familiar surroundings. I felt helpless staying in the hotel. I was depending on doctors who knew nothing about

Thomas's preexisting conditions other than what we had told them. I completed a form so the team could get Thomas's records from Everett, but all the while, I continued to wonder how I was going to get Thomas home if he was released in his current condition. He was so weak that I was not certain he could even sit up in a car for such a long ride. I did not know what to do.

At approximately 10:00 p.m. Sunday night, Thomas's temperature came down to 99.5. I stayed with him until 1:00 a.m., but the night chair in the room was uncomfortable, and the nurses' movement in and out of the room made it impossible to sleep. Though I did not know how Thomas would make the drive, I continued to hope that he would be released soon, and I knew I needed rest if that was going to happen.

"Baby, I need to go back to the hotel and get some rest. I want to be here with you, but if I'm going to drive you home, I have to get some sleep. I also want to be here in the morning when the doctors are making their rounds."

"Okay," Thomas said. "Get your rest." He showed me that he had his cell phone. "Let me know when you get back to the hotel."

I promised I would, and I left.

When I entered the hotel, I took a deep breath, then walked to the hotel desk and arranged to stay another night—to check out on Tuesday, July 25 instead of Monday as we had originally planned. We were, quite literally, taking this day by day. Everything was up in the air.

I returned to our room and began packing for the trip home. There were many leftover supplies from the reunion, as well as our clothes, that needed to be packed. Because he had not been feeling well, Thomas's clothes were all over the place, hanging on chairs and piled on the floor. Mine were not much better, having had to run back and forth from the hotel to the hospital.

When I could not keep my eyes open any longer, I went to bed. It was then I realized how lonely I was in that hotel room without Thomas.

* * *

Most of our relatives had left town by Sunday evening or were planning to leave early Monday morning. I did not see much of anyone after the banquet, but my son Michael, his wife, and his three sons were still in town.

Michael and Marna had planned to vacation in St. Simons, Georgia; my three grandbabies were going to come home with me and Thomas after the reunion. But Michael canceled that trip to St. Simons so that they would all be able to support me in Orlando and accompany me and Thomas back to Atlanta. I was so grateful.

Monday morning, July 24, brought good news. Thomas's blood pressure and temperature had been normal for nine hours. He looked like he had rounded a corner.

I left a message at the local VA office asking for assistance with Thomas's transport. A gentleman from the organization called me back and said that they had seen situations like this before where someone was sick but, in a matter of time, did not need VA assistance. So, he requested I call him back in a few days' time to ensure their services would be needed. I agreed and thanked him.

By late afternoon, however, Thomas's temperature spiked again and all he wanted to do was sleep. He did not want anybody coming in and checking on him. He complained about the hospital personnel continually "messing" with him.

And he did not want to talk to me. Thomas *always* wanted to talk to me.

Thomas's temperature fluctuated for the rest of the evening, yet every test that was conducted was negative. Blood cultures were negative. The CT scan of the thoracic region was negative. All I heard from his doctor was: "I don't know what this is."

Despite all this, I tried to maintain my optimism that we would be leaving any day. So once again, at 1:00 a.m., I left the hospital and returned to the hotel to get some sleep so that I could make the seven-hour drive when the time came. The hotel granted me another night's stay, with my checkout now scheduled for Wednesday, July 26.

* * *

When I returned to the hospital on Tuesday morning, July 25, Thomas's temperature remained high at just below 102 degrees. They performed another battery of tests—all negative, again. One of the physicians mentioned the possibility of a complication from Thomas's UTI the month prior, as there was blood in his urine.

I panicked at the mention of blood, but Dr. Chad assured me that the blood was consistent with UTI complications and that I should not worry. He still wanted Thomas's temperature to stabilize and wanted to ensure his blood was clear of infection before releasing him, but Dr. Chad said that he predicted Thomas could be discharged no earlier than Thursday, July 27.

Thomas had a physical therapy session scheduled for that morning, Tuesday, July 25, to help him regain some of his strength. The activity seemed to perk him up somewhat. He even joked with some of the nurses, and then with me. The nurse wanted Thomas to sit up in his chair for an hour that afternoon, which he did. He appeared to be far more alert and seemed to understand all the conversations with the physicians and nurses. I was hopeful that Thomas was improving, and that we would be headed home soon.

Then, sometime around noon, the hematologist arrived to tell me that Thomas was very sick. It was the first time I had actually heard someone say those words since we had arrived at the hospital. His temperature continued on the high side, and there was now an additional problem: the blood tests were indicating an infection. Thomas's platelets were dropping, and he might require a transfusion.

I did not understand what they were telling me. I did not even know what platelets were, and now they were telling me that Thomas needed a blood transfusion. He had just been sitting up in a chair and exercising with the therapist—and now he needed a transfusion? My head felt as though it was spinning on a swivel.

Later that afternoon, a nurse entered Thomas's room and said she had to perform a test for a particular virus. Without warning, she stuck a swab deep into Thomas's nose. Thomas yelled out in pain. She apologized, saying that the depth of the swab was a requirement for the test, but truthfully, she did not seem all that sorry about it. In fact, she seemed more annoyed by Thomas's reaction than anything else.

Shortly before 9:00 p.m., the test results came back.

Thomas was diagnosed with respiratory syncytial virus, or RSV, an extremely contagious virus of the respiratory tract. The nurses placed a sign on the door that indicated gowns and gloves had to be worn when entering the room, otherwise known as contact precautions. Those same gowns and gloves had to be taken off and deposited into a special receptacle before leaving the room. It all felt like a scene from some movie.

In the midst of this news, one of the staff members mentioned to me that the hospital offered hospitality rooms for people whose family members were patients in the hospital. They advised me to look into it, as they knew I was staying at a hotel and traveling back and forth at unusual hours to see Thomas. Staying in a hospitality room would be less expensive and a safer situation for me overall.

However, I decided to stay in the hotel one additional night. I still owed them money for not filling the reservation block, and hotel management had agreed that my additional nights would be applied to that obligation. They allowed me to stay one additional night, but I would have to leave on Thursday, July 27, since they had another group arriving and needed my room as part of their block.

Later that evening, on Tuesday, July 25, I received an email from the hotel sales manager that said I would not be charged for the remainder of the room shortage. They were nearly sold out for that upcoming weekend, and as a courtesy, they waived the additional charge. I guessed that the hotel administrator I had spoken to about my trips to the hospital had conveyed the message to her manager and they decided to go easy on me. Either way, it was a welcome gesture at a very difficult time, and I was grateful for their understanding and generosity.

* * *

Wednesday morning, July 26, came and, with it, more bad news. Thomas's condition was worsening and was becoming difficult to manage. The medical team told me he had developed problems with his kidneys.

This news was particularly disturbing because even though Thomas was a diabetic and on medication for his condition, he *never* had issues with his kidneys. He was tested every three to four months to ensure that his kidneys were not impacted, and he had been doing that for many years. His kidneys were fine the day we rolled him into that hospital.

That knowledge sparked a new question in my mind: *What have these people done to him?*

The team had been pumping antibiotics into him to bring down his fever, and I suspected that was having an effect on his kidneys. But no one told me that. All I kept hearing was, "We don't know."

They put Thomas on oxygen. He was delirious with fever and the nurses were using ice packs again to cool him down.

I could not believe this was happening. This was supposed to be a simple, fun trip for our family reunion, and now here we were, far away from home, far away from Thomas's doctor, while he lay there struggling and slowly deteriorating before my eyes.

Many family and friends continued their calls and texts. Some offered to help pay for my hotel or flat out give me money. They had all been so grateful for the reunion and the compilation of family stories, so now they wanted to help us in any way possible.

My heart still fills with gratitude remembering all the love and concern that flowed our way. Even though I did not answer the phone unless the call was from Michael, Tommie, or my stepdaughter Nichelle, these gestures of love meant everything to me. The texts are still on my phone to this day, and I plan to save them forever.

Despite Thomas's worsening condition, I had to figure out the logistics of checking out of the hotel the next morning. There was still so much in the room to pack, organize, and then get down to the car—leftover

T-shirts, books, souvenirs, Thomas's clothes, my clothes.

I felt so sad packing Thomas's clothes. As an ex-military man, he packed his bag in a special manner. He had a certain method of folding clothes and arranging them in such a way that they did not get wrinkled. And here I was, just throwing his things into a suitcase, hoping everything would fit.

I suddenly felt overwhelmed by it all. While I was trying to understand what was happening with Thomas, our dog was still boarded back home needing more of her special food because of her medical issues. The mail was surely piling up in our mailbox, a forthcoming special delivery required our signature, the rental SUV was overdue in regards to the return date, bills were becoming due since it was getting close to the first of the month, and I was scheduled to return to my job on Friday, July 28.

Michael and his family were still in town, but I did not want to bother them, if possible. I have always been an independent person—that has been a source of pride for me, but I think it hurt me during the time in Orlando, when I tried to manage it all. Maybe if I had let others help me shoulder the load, things could have turned out differently.

I think about that almost every day.

Thomas's doctors were talking at me—not to me—and it added to my frustration. They were not speaking in layman's terms, and the medical terminology and information only made me feel more scared and confused. Even though I tried to ask the right questions at the time, I am almost sure now that I did not.

For the first time in my life, I felt incapable of thinking on my feet with all the unknowns, the worry, and the stress. I hoped that Thomas would get better soon because I was beginning to feel like I did not have the strength to deal with even the slightest bit of bad news.

That bad news came Thursday morning, July 27, after I had packed up everything, loaded it in the SUV, and checked out of the hotel.

Thomas had been moved to the intensive care unit (ICU).

PART II

THE LOSS

CHAPTER 7

STOP TALKING TO ME LIKE A DOCTOR

I DID NOT UNDERSTAND.

"Why has he been moved to the ICU?" I asked one of the nurses. "What does that mean?"

They explained to me that he had been moved there on an "unofficial" basis. That it was not exactly the ICU, but a room on that floor that would allow him to be checked on more frequently by a team that was familiar with his situation and one that could be called upon if needed. I had never heard of an arrangement like that, but I did not question it further. I rationalized that they were a small hospital and that was just how they did things in order to stay on top of Thomas's situation.

Nearly everyone I had interacted with at Viewpark was white or a foreigner, so I later asked one of the Black nurses I befriended there if she had ever heard of an unofficial ICU stay. She said she had not, but

I thought it must have been a good thing if it meant Thomas would get more care. Still, there was always this voice, just in the background, telling me something was not right.

Had I known then what I know now.

* * *

From the moment Thomas was transferred to ICU unofficially, things got stranger and stranger. A number of different experts became involved in Thomas's care. There was a pulmonary physician, a hematology specialist, an infectious disease specialist, and a nephrologist, all coming in and out of Thomas's room during the day.

Every time they spoke to me, they used complicated medical jargon, all of it over my head. When I asked them what their opinion was, each of them, except the hematologist, would say, "From our standpoint, Mr. Brown is doing fine."

I did not understand how that could be when the hospitalist assigned to coordinate all of Thomas's care, Dr. Chad, who was also the emergency room doctor, now told me that Thomas was very, very sick. Dr. Chad explained that the specialists were only looking at the organ systems that were in their area of expertise. So, if that system seemed to be working, they would tell me he was fine, even though his overall health was poor.

It was so confusing and frustrating. I did not know what to make of it, but I tried to remain positive, choosing to find some truth in the notion that Thomas actually *was* fine.

Then, later that Thursday, July 27, the ICU physician, Dr. Zeller, said he would like to speak with me. He took me to one of the vacant rooms on the ICU floor, accompanied by a nurse.

Dr. Zeller did not bother to address me by name, which would have been a form of courtesy considering the information he was about to deliver to me. "I believe in telling it like it is," he said. There was an air of arrogance in his voice that put me on guard and made me fearful of what was to come.

"Yes, please. I agree. I need to know. We're from out of town, and I need to get back to work, and most importantly, I need to know exactly what's going on with my husband."

"Your husband is not going to make it. His kidneys have shut down, and he has issues with his blood because his bone marrow is not working. I've seen this before, and I know exactly how it's going to end."

Just like that.

Cold.

Uncaring.

Absent of any empathy.

Dr. Zeller was completely unconcerned about the impact this news would have on me. His tone and demeanor were such that it felt as though he had intended for his words to deliver the greatest possible shock to me—as if he were intentionally *trying* to shock me, *trying* to *traumatize* me.

He continued on, leaving me no time to comprehend what he had just told me. I screamed inside my head. I wanted to scream at him too, but I remembered the perception people had of Black women who act out emotionally, no matter how justified we are when we do so. I wanted nothing more than to tell this man that if my husband died, there would be a price to pay, that he would find out very quickly that he messed with the wrong person, but I restrained myself, thinking it was best not to threaten him.

Later, I could deal with Dr. Zeller, but now, I had to take care of Baby. I did not want to give them one reason to give Thomas less care than he deserved—though based on the contradictory and incomplete information I was receiving, I had a suspicion that was already occurring.

Dr. Zeller went on in more detail about Thomas's condition, not caring about my personal well-being and still, it seemed, with the intent of hurting me. I interrupted.

"Wait, wait. Just please wait one second, Doctor. Can you please call Thomas's doctor at Everett in Atlanta?"

"No," he said. "Your husband is here now."

My mouth fell open. I was shocked—then enraged. My mind raced. Does this man see *Thomas as some sort of property of his and the hospital's? Do I have no say in his care?*

"There is a problem with his bone marrow," he went on, ignoring my request. "It's not producing red blood cells properly. His breathing is labored. After a while, he's going to get tired, and eventually give up. It is possible that kidney dialysis might wake up healthy kidneys, but again, his kidneys have shut down. He is also bleeding."

I interrupted Dr. Zeller again. "Where is he bleeding?" Dr. Chad had told me Thomas had blood in his urine but not to worry. I needed to know more.

"From various places, like his mouth," he said, with absolutely zero concern in his voice.

I could not bear to hear any more. "Please, I'd like to revisit my question about you consulting with Thomas's doctor at Everett?" I pleaded, trying to remain professional and calm. *Surely*, I thought, *a patient can expect that a treating physician should acquire as much health history as possible from the patient's physician so the best possible outcomes can be achieved.*

But the doctor remained determined.

"No. I'm not going to have another doctor walking around this hospital."

I was confused and angry. "No. A telephone call," I pleaded, putting my hand to my ear like a telephone. I had told him Everett in Atlanta. He *knew* Everett was in Atlanta. Why was he talking about someone walking around his hospital? *This is so crazy!* I thought.

I could not believe how cruel Dr. Zeller was about it all. My hands trembled with fear, panic, and anger. "Well, does he have a chance?" I asked.

"He has a chance," he said coldheartedly. Dr. Zeller did not say anything further. I needed to hear more, but it seemed I would have to pull it out of him.

"Can you please explain what that means? When will we know? A week? A month?"

"A week. Not a month," he curtly said in his same cruel tone.

"I need you to call Everett," I said weakly. I was beginning to lose it.

"No," the doctor said. With that, he turned and walked away.

I broke down and began crying uncontrollably. The nurse who accompanied him to the room came over and put her arm around me—but even that felt cold, as though it was an act that she was supposed to *perform*, rather than truly consoling me. The gesture to me felt as callous as the physician she worked with.

We all left the room, and I found a chair somewhere on the ICU floor so I could get myself together. I felt so helpless. How in the world was I going to navigate a situation like this when these doctors were not truly interested in whether Thomas lived or died?

Why would Dr. Zeller refuse to talk to Thomas's doctor? Is he hiding something that he knows would be revealed if he spoke to Everett?

I was unable to focus, and my mind could not process anything more. The words that my husband was going to die echoed endlessly in my head, but I could not accept it as reality just yet.

I was in shock and traumatized. I needed to do something, *anything* to change the subject, any mundane task that I could do that did not require any real thinking and would allow me to focus on something else for a moment—so I recalled the list of things to do that I had made earlier. I ordered special food for my dog, Abby, that would be delivered to her vet where she was boarded. I called the rental car company to extend the rental period. I then called my boss, Doug, who was my direct supervisor at the time.

I was scheduled to return to work and log in the following day, Friday, July 28, though I had already informed him Thomas was not doing well in the hospital in Florida. I recall how he tried to be cheerful when answering the phone.

"Tell me some good news, Jonnie."

It was difficult to talk without getting emotional. "No, Doug. I've been told that Thomas isn't going to make it." I explained that I did not know what the future held right now, and then I asked for an additional week off.

"I'm so sorry, Jonnie. Anything you need. Take as much time as you need. Just keep me posted."

Back in 2013, when my mother's health started to decline, I began teleworking. Both Melissa and Doug were so gracious in approving my request for permanent telework then, just as Doug was gracious about giving me time off now.

After getting off the phone with Doug, I called Tommie and told her about Dr. Zeller's conversation. I told her that she had to come to Orlando *now*—I could not do this anymore by myself. I had been keeping her abreast of Thomas's condition all along, and she was very upset at hearing this latest development.

I gave Tommie my credit card information and told her to book a flight and come right away, no matter how much the cost. She later texted me her flight information. She would arrive on Saturday evening, July 29.

Michael and his family were still in town taking in the Orlando attractions. The boys were not allowed to come into the ICU, so Michael and Marna were keeping them entertained while trying to be supportive to me. Michael would visit Thomas while I would visit with Michael's wife and children in common areas of the hospital, where the boys were allowed. I still tried to not disrupt their activities and burden them, but I know now I should have asked Michael in no uncertain terms for his help in figuring all of this out.

After I talked to them, Marna called her father, a physician in Oakland, California. He briefly spoke with me about Thomas's condition, but I still was not clear on what direct steps I should take at that point.

I also kept Nichelle updated about Thomas's condition, so she was already on her way to Orlando, arriving around midnight on Thursday, July 27. I shared Dr. Zeller's conversation with her, and she broke down and cried. I explained how she needed to suit up in a gown and gloves before entering Thomas's room and to take them off when exiting. Thomas had been given pain medication so, sadly, I am not sure if he even knew that Nichelle was at his bedside.

I had a terrible time sleeping that Thursday night in the hospitality suite. I was so scared to lose my husband. I knew I had to be strong and prepare for his death at any moment, yet at the same time, I wanted to have hope that he could pull through. That meant I had to do everything I could to help him. Thomas always took care of me, and now it was my turn to take care of him.

I did not know how I would manage being alone after forty-five years with this wonderful man. I was not ready.

* * *

The next day, when I was at Thomas's bedside, I noticed Dr. Zeller standing right outside Thomas's doorway. He was not looking into Thomas's room, and the layout of the floor was such that it was obvious his stop there was purposeful. He stood motionless in front of the glass door, as if waiting for me to notice his profile.

It was strange. Dr. Zeller had been walking down the hallway, but he chose to stop right there at Thomas's room, doing nothing. It reminded me of a gangster scene in a movie, as though his presence was a warning of some kind. I turned my back on him and gave my attention to Thomas. The thought of speaking to that doctor again was simply unbearable, and I did not want to look at him.

Looking back, I have tried to figure out why he stopped there. I believe this was a form of passive intimidation, to stop me from trying to get them to consult with Thomas's doctor at Everett.

I think it is because they knew they had done something wrong.

* * *

I never told Thomas that he was going to die.

Back in 2012, when my father was nearing his ninety-seventh birthday, he became very ill after developing aspiration pneumonia. His doctor told me that it was time for him to go to hospice. My father had directly asked me if he was going to make it, but I did not know what to say.

"Daddy, you've had pneumonia before. You are so strong, and you've always pulled through before." I never actually answered his question, and I carried a great deal of guilt about that afterward.

When I asked Thomas if I should have told my father that he was not going to live, Thomas thought about it for a while. Then he looked at me and said, "No."

He said nothing else. Simply "no."

I remembered that conversation as I thought about whether or not to tell Thomas how grave his situation was—and decided I would not tell him. It was hard to make that decision and much harder yet to pretend that nothing was wrong.

I had to deal with how I was feeling about losing my husband, but then I also had to try to keep myself together so I could listen to what these doctors were telling me and ensure I made the best decisions. All the while, whenever I was with Thomas, I had to pretend that nothing was wrong. Selfishly, I was glad for the times he was sleeping, because I did not have to put on the act.

I felt like three different people—one for Thomas, one for the doctors, and one for myself. This constant metamorphosis I found myself going through was exhausting and overwhelming. I felt like I had no control over anything, which was a situation that I seldom experienced before.

Before he got sick, Thomas often would say to me, "Can you just relax? You're always thinking about something. You need to slow down and enjoy the here and now." That was how my mind worked—except now that he was sick, it was not working at all. My brain was a hamster on a wheel, thoughts just going around and around and around. I could not properly process information. I could not get a handle on anything going on. I could not think straight.

Later, I learned that I was probably in a state of severe emotional shock because of this life-changing event and the way in which it was presented to me. I had experienced a rush of overwhelming emotions, which I was not ready to understand or respond to. My brain was unable to process the situation, and it froze to protect my mind and body.

* * *

On Friday, July 28, the doctors informed me that Thomas was not voiding any urine and that they were going to attempt dialysis to see if they could revive his kidney function. I encouraged Thomas to urinate in the urinal they had provided, but he could not. With all of that buildup in his kidneys, dialysis was the only choice.

After I left Thomas's bedside sometime that day, a tube was inserted into the jugular vein in his neck. I suppose the staff knew to wait until I was gone because I could not watch that being done.

When I came back, I noticed Thomas's right arm, where the IV had been inserted, was red and swollen. I brought it to the attention of Dr. Hamilton, who was filling in for Dr. Chad.

"Yes, it's infected," he said. "It's okay. We don't need to worry about it."

Yet another of what was becoming a series of brush-offs. Things had gone so terribly wrong, but no one was telling me much.

Despite that awful news, I took note of how nice Thomas's hair looked on the pillow. His hair was fairly straight with big natural waves in it. I remembered asking him years ago what he did to his hair to make that big Afro he wore when I first met him. He just said, playfully, "Ah, you don't know, do you?" I think he used bar soap or something harsh like that to make his hair frizz up—but he never did tell me.

Thomas had recently allowed my hairdresser and neighbor, Cynthia, to cut his hair. He had difficulty finding someone who could cut his wavy hair correctly so that it would lay down on his head, but he was pleased with how Cynthia cut it. She had most recently cut his hair just before the family reunion. I texted Cynthia. "Your haircut is kickin' it on the pillow." It was a nice moment in the midst of all that terribleness.

Thomas had his first dialysis session that afternoon. I was told that the next twenty-four to forty-eight hours afterward were going to be critical to Thomas's survival. I do not do well in hospitals to begin with, but I made the mistake of looking into the room as Thomas was undergoing dialysis. Thomas's head shook as blood pumped through the tube coming through his neck. It upset me so much to see him that way that I had to leave.

Later that evening, I stepped away from Thomas's room to get something to eat in the cafeteria. When I returned, I discovered they had inserted a feeding tube into Thomas's stomach. Earlier, the doctors had told me that Thomas was weak, so I asked them when they were going to feed him. No one had ever told me that he was having swallowing difficulties or that they were going to step up to a feeding tube.

It occurred to me that there was a pattern forming. Whenever I left the room, they performed some new procedure on Thomas—most recently, the insertion of the port for his dialysis or the feeding tube. It was clear they were watching me, waiting for their opportunity to do these things to my husband when I was not present. At the time, I chalked it up to the idea that they thought I would not be able to handle seeing it, or that seeing these procedures would upset me too much. But now I am not sure what to think.

Nichelle said on Friday, July 28 that we needed to take Thomas back to Atlanta, back to Everett. When she said it, I immediately thought, *She's right. That's what we need to do.* I cannot say why that notion had not occurred to me sooner, but as I said, my mind had betrayed me in the midst of all this chaos—in particular, after the conversation with Dr. Zeller when he said Thomas was not going to live. As soon as Nichelle said, "Take him back," I started working on how I was going to make that happen.

I spoke to Dr. Hamilton again, the physician who was filling in for Dr. Chad, and told him that I wanted to move Thomas home to be cared for by his own doctors. He said he would pass that information on to the "folks who could help you do that." As in my previous conversations with him, he essentially passed the buck, as if to say, "Look, I'm just the covering physician here. This is someone else's problem, not mine."

I called my health insurance company to see if there was any way they would cover the transport from Viewpark Hospital to Everett. From a previous experience involving Michael, I knew the odds were slim, because if there were facilities in the area that could provide the necessary care, insurance would not pay for the transport home—but I wanted to confirm with my insurance regardless. I had to get Thomas out of there.

Sure enough, BCBS told me what I already knew, so I was not upset. I would make that transport happen regardless.

* * *

After three days of being off duty, Dr. Chad was back in the hospital on Saturday, July 29—and he brought more bad news.

He informed me that Thomas was bleeding somewhere in the stomach area. He did not know exactly where, but Thomas was, according to Dr. Chad, too ill for them to perform an endoscopy. Ironically, the procedure was the only way for them to identify the source of the bleeding so that it could be repaired.

When Thomas came to this hospital, his kidneys were fine, and he was not bleeding. I got so upset thinking about all the things these doctors had done to destroy Thomas's health. I asked Dr. Chad about Thomas's arm with the IV and the possible infection.

"It's not infected," he said. "It's a blood clot."

"A blood clot?"

"Yes, but that's the least of my worries."

It was frightening to think that a clot in Thomas's arm could be the least of his worries, but Dr. Chad went on to tell me that he had to assess the risks of Thomas's bleeding versus the risk of the clot moving to his heart. He felt that ignoring the clot was less of a risk than everything else that was going on with Thomas, so he did nothing about the arm. Nothing.

On what was becoming one of the rare occasions when Thomas was alert, he slowly lifted that arm to look at it. He held it there for as long as he could, looking it up and down. Then he lowered it back down to the bed, closed his eyes, and let out a deep and resigned sigh. That sigh said everything. Baby knew he was in bad shape.

I tried to ask the doctors what I thought were the right questions, but I did not know what to do with the answers. Family members know that when a loved one is in the hospital, we must stay with them for twenty-four hours a day to ensure that we are aware of everything that is going on—but what may be learned is almost meaningless if we do not have the medical background to interpret what is being said.

It seemed that every bit of information that the various specialists relayed to me was filled with complicated medical jargon. They would say things to me that I still have trouble pronouncing. I got so frustrated at one point that after one of the specialists left the room, I went out to the nurse's station and banged my fist on the desk.

"You all have got to do better than this!" I shouted. "These doctors are coming in here and talking to me like I'm one of them. Stop talking to me like a doctor!"

It was like shouting into the wind. No one cared. These people were called in to "consult." Once that was done, they were gone. It seemed like Thomas represented an invoice to them, not a person whose condition required thought and evaluation. It seemed Dr. Chad viewed Thomas the same way as well.

One doctor, a hematologist assigned to Thomas, was a bit friendlier than her counterparts, and I felt comfortable asking her questions because she was willing to provide answers and explain using layman's terms. She told me how sick Thomas was based on all of his blood tests.

"What are you looking at?" I asked. "What is it you're seeing that I can't see when I look at my husband?"

She took me over to her computer and showed me the levels of Thomas's platelet count or hematocrit. She told me what his levels were when he entered the hospital, what they were now, and what the normal range should be. What I learned from her is that Thomas's platelets had continued to drop, which explained the bleeding he was experiencing because platelets help the blood to clot.

But I also learned that no one was doing anything about it.

I also told Dr. Chad that I wanted to transfer Thomas to Everett. He explained the process to me, what he called a doctor-to-doctor transfer. He would be responsible for initiating conversations with an Everett emergency physician to share information about Thomas's condition. The hospital would transmit medical records to Everett so that their physicians would be able to immediately run with Thomas's care upon arrival. I would be responsible for making payment for the cost of the emergency transport, and there were people on staff that could help with arranging that transportation.

Then, in a patronizing and condescending tone, Dr. Chad said, "You know all of that costs a lot of money, don't you?"

That made me so unbelievably annoyed. His tone. The way he said what he said. *These doctors in this hospital are so disrespectful to the patients and their families,* I thought. Dr. Chad would have never said that to a white person. He would not have even said that to a *poor* white person because he would have assumed they might know another white person with the financial means to deliver the money.

But with a Black woman standing in front of him, he assumed I could not *possibly* have knowledge about emergency transportation costs and, more specifically, that I could not *possibly* have the means to pay for it. Yes, I was in the same clothes I had been wearing the last few days, but they were all I had. Yes, I was wearing my worn comfortable shoes—the shoes I drive in, so I do not scuff the heels of my good shoes—but that should not have mattered. He had no right to speak to me that way.

I knew full well that the transfer would cost thousands of dollars. I also knew there was no price I would not pay for Thomas's care. I just wanted him out of this hospital and back home where he belonged.

I took a step toward Dr. Chad and looked him dead in the eye.

"Don't you worry about the money. You just take care of the doctor-to-doctor transfer, and I'll handle the rest."

With that, I turned my back on him and walked away.

* * *

Thomas had his second dialysis session Saturday, July 29, and while I was told it went well, we were still in a "wait and see" frame of mind. Afterward, I spoke to the nephrologist, who told me that Thomas's health was declining and that his body was not handling all the stress well. He also said that Thomas's blood pressure was dropping, and a stroke or heart attack could come at any time.

Yet no one told me what it was that was causing all of this. I never got a picture from anyone as to what exactly was going on with Thomas. Everyone seemed to be operating in their own silo. All I wanted to do was get Thomas out of there so that I could deal with professionals who knew what they were doing and who understood the importance of properly communicating with family members—the kind of communication that Thomas and I always experienced at teaching and research hospitals and at the clinics where we always received our healthcare.

In the meantime, Thomas was dying in slow motion, right in front of me. I later likened it to the murder of George Floyd. I watched George Floyd slowly lose his life, crying for help from the people that were supposed to protect and serve him—and received none. Thomas and I were also crying for help from those with the knowledge and know-how to save a life. Our insurance paid a lot of money for us to receive the proper help—but we received none.

It was a challenge to control my anger, but I knew the minute I acted in ways they found the least bit unprofessional that they would have seen me as the hysterical angry Black woman. I would not give them that satisfaction, nor would I give them any excuse to treat us any worse than they already were, despite how disrespected I felt.

Our lives did not matter to them. We were nobody.

Sunday made that painfully clear.

CHAPTER 8

ALIVE, ALONE, AND DIRTY

MICHAEL AND HIS FAMILY LEFT SATURDAY, JULY 29, AS MICHAEL had to return to work on Monday and the kids had to get back to school. He knew my sister would be in town that evening to support me, so they got on the road that night and returned to their home in Texas.

First thing on Sunday morning, July 30, my sister and I headed to the ICU floor. The attendant at the desk buzzed us into the unit. There was a long, wide hallway to get to Thomas's room.

There was no one at the nurses' station. There were no lights turned on, but daylight was streaming in through the windows. My first thought was that Thomas had died during the early morning after I left him.

We rushed to his room. At the same time, I was holding my breath. My heart raced with the anticipation that we would get there and find it empty.

Thomas was there, but he was alone in the room, filthy as can be—and it was clear he had been like that for a while. He had pulled out his feeding tube, and the liquid had spread all over him, caked and dried to the sheets. His gown was crumpled and dirty, and the sheets had been pulled from the corners of the mattress as though he had been writhing and thrashing in the night. His mouth hung open, and his breathing was labored. His sheets were stained by his bloody stools.

Was he experiencing pain?

They left him there all alone. On a unit where he was supposed to be watched closely. In the unofficial ICU.

I was so upset, and I did not know what to do. I momentarily paced back and forth in disbelief that they had done this—that they would leave him like this with no one to monitor him. My sister was just as upset and angry.

I heard sounds out in the hallway. A nurse had arrived at the nurses' station. I immediately approached her.

"Are you here to take care of my husband, Thomas Brown?"

She said she was. The nurse was a Black woman, and I wanted to connect with her in the hopes that maybe someone could help us through all of this.

"Are you an employee or a contractor?" I asked. I did not trust the people who were employed at this hospital anymore, and I needed to know her relationship to the hospital.

"I'm a contractor."

I grabbed her hand, and I broke down and cried.

"Please help me. Please. Please help us."

She held my hand back and asked me what was wrong—and it all came pouring out. I told her all of it: that my husband came here with cold symptoms but was now very sick, that all I wanted to do was get him back home to his doctors. That they left him here all by himself, to lay in filth for who knows how long.

"Don't worry," she said. "I'll take care of him." Her name was Frances.

Frances got to work. She called for someone to come help her. Another nurse arrived, and they put on their protective equipment and entered the room. Frances was about to exit Thomas's room at one point, but she stopped short and spoke to me. I was standing outside of his room without any protective equipment.

"Mrs. Brown, I can't keep going in and out of the room, putting on and taking off my gloves and gown. Do you mind helping me?"

"Tell me what you want me to do," I said. "I'll do anything."

Thomas apparently was not important enough for the hospital to send the proper help that was needed to take care of him. Because only one other nurse came to help her, Frances needed *me* to get her the supplies necessary to clean up Thomas and his bed. *I* went to the oven to get warm cloths so that she could wipe him down. *I* brought her the clean sheets to change out.

"I'm so sorry," Frances told me. "This hospital just doesn't care about Black people. I've seen similar situations to this so many times when it comes to Black patients. If I had been here overnight, I would have done my best to take care of your husband. You need to get your husband out of this hospital."

She later told me that once, while she was caring for Thomas, he took her hand in his.

"He wasn't able to talk, but he communicated with me through eye contact and the squeezing of my hand. I remember that look in his eyes as he laid in the hospital bed, so weak that he wasn't able to do anything for himself.

"That was how your husband said thank you."

I lost it. I could not hold back the tears.

* * *

That afternoon, a discharge nurse approached me with information about two quotes she had gotten for the medical transport to Everett. One was for Tuesday, August 1, for $8,700 and one on Wednesday, August 2 for approximately $3,800. I told her that I wanted the one leaving Tuesday as I wanted him out of there as soon as possible, more than ever. She gave me the paperwork and I completed it.

The discharge nurse also told me that she had to get a pre-certification from my health insurance in order to transfer Thomas to Everett, and that this process would take approximately two days. She left before I could ask her why it would take that long, let alone why pre-certification was needed in the first place. I had a premium health insurance plan, one that did not require preapproval for anything except elective surgery.

I decided to call BCBS myself to expedite matters. Two days to make a telephone call? *How ridiculous*, I thought. *Time is of the essence.*

"Oh, no, Mrs. Brown," the BCBS representative said. "You don't need a pre-certification at all. Just like you walked into the emergency department at Viewpark Hospital or walked into emergency at Everett, you can fly into emergency at Everett, and you do not need a pre-certification."

At that exact moment, the discharge nurse walked back into the room.

"Mrs. Brown," she said in a loud voice. "There are too many hands in the pot. I'm trying to get a hold of BCBS, and they're telling me that they're talking to you right now."

For a moment, I stared at her. *You told me it was going to take two days,* I thought, *and now you're standing here yelling at me because I'm on the phone, trying to get quicker answers, and you're telling me there are too many hands in the pot?*

I felt the pressure in my head building. I took a breath and then handed her my phone.

"Well, here's the lady from BCBS. Take care of it, please. Right now."

She took the phone from me and spoke with the representative. When she hung up, I asked her if she had the information she needed, because I was told I did *not* need a pre-certification to transfer Thomas at all. She begrudgingly said yes. So, the issue she told me was going to take two days to resolve was taken care of in less than five minutes.

I could not help but wonder, *Don't they have competent personnel who deal with enough patients and their insurance companies to know the various insurance plans, especially my premier health plan from the federal government?* Every place Thomas and I had ever gone to for care immediately recognized the quality of our health plan. Why would they tell me it takes two days to find out how my insurance works when we had just walked into this very hospital a week ago, when they probably rushed to confirm with BCBS that my insurance would cover Thomas's care? Even if Everett did require pre-certification, BCBS was always ready and available to immediately confirm that. This entire interaction over insurance was puzzling, to say the least. But it was resolved now, and I had other things to worry about.

Later that day, I was happy to see Thomas awake and alert. At that time, Nichelle and Tommie were both in the room too. He pointed at each of them and said, "You're here? And you're here?"

They told him they were there to see him and to help him get well. They knew I had not told Thomas that he was going to die.

Thomas was ready to leave the hospital. He pointed to Nichelle and asked, "You're ready to go?"

"Yeah," she said.

Then he pointed to Tommie. "Are you ready to go?"

"Yes," she said.

He looked at me. "Everybody's ready to go, Jonnie. So, get me my shoes."

"Baby," I said. "We're working on a medical transport to get you back to Everett."

"Jonnie, please just take me home and let me lay in my chair. I promise to go to the doctor tomorrow."

My heart broke when he said that. His voice was just so pitiful and pleading, and he was making a promise to me. He loved that recliner chair so much, and he spent so much time in it. That I could not take him home right then and there was almost too much to bear.

Thomas told us he was thirsty. I put a little bit of water on a sponge and rubbed it on his tongue and lips. I had been instructed by the nurse to do this because he had forgotten how to swallow and his doctors were afraid he would aspirate, or let the water into his lungs. This was the first I heard of swallowing issues.

Thomas did not like the sponge and got frustrated with me and raised his voice asking for water. By the sound of his voice, I could tell his tongue was thickening. I saw his gums were bleeding. I reported this to Dr. Chad, who told me that Thomas was doing poorly and bleeding internally, but that he was still too sick to have an endoscopy to determine the issue.

It was at this point that I began to question transferring Thomas to Everett. I was worried the trip itself might kill him. Or were his chances better here? I did not know what to do.

Thomas had another round of dialysis that afternoon. During that time, Nichelle checked out of her hotel room since she was able to get a hospitality room at the hospital as well. Many of my cousins and friends continued to call and text that day, wanting to help in any way they could, especially giving us money. Though I knew they were only trying to love me and help me, I got somewhat frustrated with their insistence—my mind was stretched so thin. But no matter how many times I told them we were fine, their love and concern for us would not take no for an answer.

Finally, I relented and asked my cousin Darryl to set up a GoFundMe page to raise money for the air transportation to Everett. The outpouring of support was simply incredible. Everyone prayed for

Thomas and asked their congregations to do the same. I was overwhelmed by their generosity and how much money had been raised in a short amount of time.

I stayed with Thomas until about 5:00 a.m. the next morning, Monday, July 31, until I just could not stay awake any longer. In fact, I dozed off more than once, but the activity on the floor frequently woke me. I was so tired and just wanted to go to my room, but I feared leaving Thomas alone, thinking that the nurses would abandon him once again or that he might die without me.

I was incensed thinking about this predicament. It was hard enough to worry about Thomas. Why did I also have to worry about whether the medical personnel would abandon him or whether they would properly tend to him? It was too much to think about, and my mind just could not take on any more problems. So, I stayed there as long as I could.

When I could not keep my eyes open any longer, I went to my room to get a few hours of sleep. I did not want to be away from Thomas any more than that, so when I woke, I quickly prepped my bags so that I could leave in a hurry if need be. I knew once we got word that Thomas could be airlifted, he would be gone, and since I would not be permitted to ride with him, I had to be ready to jump in the car and make the seven-hour drive to Atlanta or catch a plane—if the flight and the time spent in airports was less than seven hours.

I was ready to bring Thomas home.

* * *

Later that morning, Monday, July 31, after a few hours of sleep, I rushed to the ICU floor to find Dr. Chad standing outside Thomas's room. I rushed up to him, panicked and out of breath.

"Dr. Chad, do you have the doctor-to-doctor transfer, do you have the transfer?"

He looked at me blankly but did not respond right away.

"You need to call," he said to me, coldly.

"Wait a second. You explained to me yesterday that that was a call *you* had to make—that *you* had to speak to the doctor and make the arrangements."

He said it again, emotionless, "You need to call."

I was confused—and incensed. Why was it so difficult to communicate with these people? This made absolutely no sense.

I went to Thomas's room, dumbfounded. As I stood there, I tried to think of all the reasons why Dr. Chad might have told me that I needed to call. Maybe he had difficulty navigating the Everett system which, after all, was a big hospital.

But intuitively I knew that was not the issue.

All of these people in this hospital seemed determined to throw obstacles in front of me. There was no desire to help me at all. In fact, they blocked me from every direction when I tried to get the help my husband needed. At every turn, I experienced more emotional stress, so it is no wonder why I continued to have difficulty thinking.

I knew the Everett Primary Care appointment line by memory. I felt I could not wait even a second to look up any other number, so I pulled out my phone and called them. When the woman came on the line, I was crying, and I begged her to help me.

"My name is Jonnie Brown. My husband's name is Thomas Brown. We are long-standing patients at Everett. Please help me. We're in Florida, and I have to get him home to Everett. He's very sick. Please help me. Please." The woman was sympathetic, and I could tell she was on the verge of tears, too, hearing my pleas.

"Mrs. Brown. You called the Primary Care appointment line. I don't know what to do. But please hold on, and I'll find someone to help you."

In less than a minute, another woman came on the line. Her tone was authoritative yet kind.

"Mrs. Brown, I'm going to help you. I don't know what to do, either, but please stay on the line because I'm going to find out how to help you. It might take five minutes. It might take ten. Please hold on until I come back to the call."

I continued to cry, despite—or perhaps because of—her willingness to help. I felt so trapped in this hospital, where no one seemed to care at all about Thomas or me, that the simple act of someone saying they were going to help me meant so much.

The woman finally returned to the line.

"Mrs. Brown, you want to speak to the Nursing and Transfer Services Department. Here is the number in case we get disconnected. When I transfer you, ask to speak to a woman by the name of Martha, in case she's not the one to answer the phone. I've already spoken to her about your situation."

She completed the transfer, and I was connected with Martha. I repeated everything I had originally told the Primary Care staff when she gently stopped me mid-sentence.

"Mrs. Brown, I'm sorry, but you can't do this. This has to be done with a doctor-to-doctor transfer."

It was then that I realized that Dr. Chad had sent me on a wild goose chase. For what reason, I still did not understand. I thanked Martha, hung up, and marched out to the nurse's station.

"Call Dr. Chad," I told them in a tone that told them I was not to be trifled with. "Get him back here *now*."

He must have been nearby, because within moments of my request, he appeared in front of me.

"Here is the number to Everett," I said. "I need you to call them right now. And I need to listen."

To my surprise, he put up no resistance. He walked me to the phone outside Thomas's room and dialed the number.

I wish I had asked him to put the call on speakerphone—but I did not think about that at the time. However, I heard his side of the call. When Everett picked up, he announced who he was and that he was calling to transfer a patient from Viewpark Hospital to Everett. The person at Everett asked for Thomas's birthday, and I provided Dr. Chad with that information. It was clear that the person on the line also asked about Thomas's condition. Dr. Chad rattled off five conditions: melena, kidney injury, RSV, bronchitis, on two liters of oxygen. There was some additional back and forth between him and the Everett representative. It was also clear Dr. Chad did not like what he was being told—he appeared to be even more disinterested than when he began the call. He answered some additional questions, then hung up.

"They'll give me a call when they get in touch with his physician."

With that, Dr. Chad walked away, leaving me standing there, gripped by anticipation and anxiety. We were so close. He had made the call to Everett, but the wait to hear back would be excruciating. Still, it was the closest to good news we had had in days.

It would be the last such news.

* * *

Thomas became more and more agitated that Monday night and into Tuesday morning, August 1. He would not sleep. He pulled off his monitoring devices. He kicked off the boots protecting his heels and legs from developing bedsores. Whenever he did these things, it took an inordinate amount of time for the nurses to come check on him, and put his monitoring devices back on, despite the fact that he had been moved to this ICU floor so the team could respond quickly to his needs.

That was a lie. Thomas simply was not a priority for them.

When he tried for the second time to remove his monitors, I reached for his hand in an attempt to stop him. He grabbed my wrist and squeezed it hard. He looked at me with eyes I had never seen before. Thomas had never laid a hand on me, and the force with which he did so now startled me. He was nonverbal at this point, but I could see in his face that he just wanted to be left alone—for me to leave him alone. This time, tears rolled down my face as I let him remove his monitoring devices. I did not want to agitate him even more than what he was. I wondered how long it would take for a nurse to check on him this time.

They never did. I had to leave the room to find someone to help.

Thomas's breathing became more and more labored. He was wearing himself out, just like Dr. Zeller had told me he would do. It was so hard to watch him go through it all.

At approximately 3:00 a.m., a nurse came to the room and told me they were receiving updates from Everett every twelve hours about the availability of an ICU bed there and that there were still no ICU beds available at that time. Thomas was resting better at that time, so I returned to my room to try to get a couple hours of sleep, hoping that Thomas would be transferred to Everett soon and I would be on my way to Atlanta. This was all so emotionally exhausting, and I looked forward to sleeping to give myself a mental break.

On Tuesday morning, August 1, Tommie, Nichelle, and I hurried to Thomas's room as quickly as we could, hoping for word about the transfer to Everett. As we approached his room, the technician responsible for his kidney dialysis that morning was removing his gown and exiting the room. He spoke to a nurse outside the room—not to me—to say that the nephrologist had instructed him to stop dialysis.

I will make no secret of the fact that I did not care for this nurse, Mable. For the entirety of our stay, she always spoke to me in the most distasteful manner, as though she had a chip on her shoulder for even having to deal with me and Thomas in the first place. Was she having a bad day everyday?

Mable walked up to me after speaking with the dialysis technician.

"Thomas's blood is bad," she said.

"What does that mean?"

As if on cue, Dr. Chad walked up to join us.

"Mrs. Brown, Mr. Brown's condition is worsening. His kidneys have shut down, as you know, but now all of his other organs are beginning to shut down, and we don't want him to be in pain. We should do everything we can to make him comfortable.

"He should go to hospice."

CHAPTER 9

YOU PROMISED TO DO NO HARM

Nichelle, Tommie, and I stood there, stunned.

This was the news I had dreaded. The news I had tried—but failed—to prepare myself for.

It was the end for Thomas, the end of our life together. I thought about how Thomas had told me on several occasions that he did not want to be a burden to anyone, that he only wanted to live as long as he could thrive and take care of himself.

In light of that, I had to ask myself, *Do I continue to fight because it's difficult for me to face the moment? Or do I accept the fact that Thomas is dying and that he needs to be made comfortable? Do I still try to move him to Everett? What if the move causes him to die on the way there?*

We still had not gotten notice that there was an ICU bed available at Everett. Thomas's kidneys had failed. His other organs were shutting down, according to Dr. Chad. He could have a stroke or a heart attack at any time.

What would Thomas say if he could tell me what to do?

I tried as best I could to recall all the information the medical team had given me, including the confusing information I had received from all of the specialists, the ones who said from their perspective that Thomas was doing fine. Yet Dr. Chad consistently told me Thomas was doing poorly, despite the reports from the specialists. And now he was telling me Thomas had to go to hospice. My head was swimming with conflicting thoughts. I just wanted someone who was committed to saving Thomas's life to tell me what to do, to help me make a decision.

Tommie and Nichelle said nothing. They waited to see what I would say. I wanted Thomas to be comfortable. I did not want him to suffer any longer.

"Okay," I finally said. "Thomas needs peace. And so do I."

Nichelle started crying and walked away. Tommie stayed rooted to her spot. I walked up to Dr. Chad and pointed a finger in his face.

"You promised," I said, crying. "You promised."

He looked at me, puzzled.

"You promised to do no harm."

I continued talking to him, rambling really, about how I felt about the medical care received. I cannot remember how Dr. Chad reacted to what I said, but Tommie did. She told me the minute I called him out regarding his oath, his head dropped. He was visibly shaken.

I pressed on, telling him that I knew that the nurse was present to be a witness when he told me about Thomas's condition. I told them how unhappy I was with the medical treatment and the care that Thomas received and their horrible bedside manner. I told him that the patient and the family's mental well-being was just as important as the medical care, and that they had completely neglected it all. "And that guy right there," I pointed to Dr. Zeller, who was across the floor, "has not heard the last from me."

Dr. Chad asked, "Who?" as he spun around.

"That guy right there." I pointed again at Dr. Zeller.

I told them it was apparent that they just did not care about us. Dr. Chad said nothing, and neither did the nurse. In fact, I looked her dead in the eyes when I spoke about the lack of bedside manner—and she stared back, as if locked in some competition with me.

I would not be the one to break eye contact, not that day. I told myself that I would keep talking until she looked away. I had had enough, and it was her turn to give in—not mine. Finally, she averted her eyes.

But that was an insignificant battle to win amid a war I had lost. I still did not know what had happened to my husband, and now he was dying. That's when it hit me.

"Where are Thomas's medical records?" I asked Dr. Chad.

From the time Thomas entered the emergency department, I had been requesting copies of Thomas's medical records, never to receive them. I did not press every day for the records because I understood it would be more efficient to give me the entire file when we left the hospital. Now, I planted my feet firmly on the floor and crossed my arms. "I'm not leaving this hospital until I get my husband's medical records." My body language and tone made it clear that I was not to be trifled with, not in that moment or going forward.

"We'll get them for you," Dr. Chad said, quietly. Then he abruptly handed me a form on a clipboard. "This is a 'do not resuscitate' order we'll need you to sign." His face was blank. Emotionless. He didn't ask me to sit down or if I had questions or about how I felt about this decision—we just stood outside Thomas's room.

I was mentally and emotionally exhausted. I did not want Thomas to suffer, so I signed the order and handed it back to Dr. Chad. He instructed the nurse to get me the records and then left the area.

Not long after, two more nurses entered the room. They removed Thomas's IV. They disconnected him from the monitoring devices. They removed his feeding tube.

I stood there and watched as they prepared my husband to die.

It was too much to bear as I moved closer to Thomas. How had this all happened? I placed one hand on his arm and the other on his chest and just stared at him. His eyes were closed. He had been in and out of consciousness, and while he slept, he looked so peaceful.

"I love you, Baby," I told him, tears rolling down my face.

An hour or so later, two women from the hospice team arrived with additional paperwork for me to fill out and all kinds of questions to answer. I did so, almost on autopilot, as though my hands and mouth moved on their own. A few more hours passed, and two men came to the room with a gurney to transport Thomas to hospice.

They were so careless with his body. They swung him onto the gurney like a rag doll, and I wondered how many more insults we would have to bear.

"Please take care with my husband."

"Yes, ma'am," they said with a dismissive tone. It was clear they felt Thomas was just another dying body. Nothing new to them.

Everything to me.

I accompanied Thomas through the hospital and outside to an emergency medical transport and inside the vehicle on the ride to hospice. I told him I loved him the whole way while I rubbed his hand and arm. Over and over again, "I love you, Baby. I love you."

At one point, the transport hit a bump, and Thomas opened his eyes. He turned his head toward me and stared at me, his kind, smiling eyes now filled with sadness and dullness.

"I remember what you told me, Baby," I said. "I know what you want." I was referring to the fact that I was trying to honor his wish of how he wanted to live.

Thomas turned his head away and closed his eyes for the rest of the trip.

It was the last time I would see his beautiful hazel eyes.

* * *

After a thirty-minute ride, we arrived at the hospice facility at approximately 3:00 p.m. While many people today choose to stay home for their hospice care, this one was part of the hospital system, on the fourth floor of one of their larger regional hospitals.

The men wheeled Thomas into the building, and I followed along, distraught. It all still seemed so surreal to me. We had come to Orlando for a happy occasion, and I was going to return home without the love of my life.

My sister and stepdaughter arrived in another vehicle shortly after. The team took Thomas to his assigned room, and a staff member came to me in the reception area to take my information. When she left, a physician appeared, and she began to discuss Thomas's condition with me while we stood there.

Do any of these people sit down with the family to make them comfortable while discussing these difficult situations? I wondered.

I told the physician I did not want Thomas to suffer and to please make him comfortable.

"How long does he have?" I asked.

The doctor was somber. "Twenty-four to thirty-six hours."

She asked us to wait while they got Thomas situated in his room. As soon as they were done, we would be able to see him.

When we entered his room, Thomas lay there peacefully. They had tucked him in tight with his hands under the covers. There was an oxygen tube in his nose that made a faint whistle as he breathed. The room had a peaceful and calm ambiance. The three of us sat together with Thomas.

After talking with each other for a while, we realized that we had not eaten anything all day. We decided to go to the cafeteria in the building. After returning to Thomas's room, Tommie said that she needed to go back to the hospitality suite at Viewpark Hospital to rest. She needed a break from it all. It had been such a shock to us, and Tommie had just recovered from a bout of shingles and feared the stress would cause her to relapse. We told the hospice team we would be leaving but would soon return.

When we arrived back at Viewpark, I informed the woman in charge of the hospitality rooms of Thomas's situation, as well as the doctor's prognosis. I told her I would inform her as soon as he passed and asked if we were allowed to stay in the hospitality suite as long as Thomas was a patient of the system. I asked if I had to leave the moment he passed or if I was allowed to stay the night so I could leave the next morning for the drive home. She told me to spend the night, by all means, so that we could rest before getting back on the road. It felt so odd and frightening and sad to make these plans, but there we were. There was no other choice.

We all returned to hospice around 11:00 p.m. We were all dreading going back and facing the inevitable, but we knew we had to get back to support Thomas. An hour or so passed before my sister finally said she could not stay any longer.

"I can't do this, Jonnie. I'm so sorry. I just can't do this. It's too much."

That is when Nichelle spoke up.

"I can't stay either."

Earlier, when Tommie and I were alone, she confided in me that despite how strong Nichelle had seemed, she had broken down when I was not around, to the point where she nearly collapsed. Tommie had to hold her up to keep her from hitting the ground. Knowing that, when she told me that she could not stay either, I understood.

"I understand," I told them. "But I'm staying. I'm not going to leave Thomas alone."

They left just before midnight. I decided to take some pictures of Thomas. I stood over him and touched his face and his chest.

"Baby, I'm so sorry," I cried. "I'm so, so sorry." I said it over and over again, unable to stop crying. "I'm sorry I couldn't protect you. I'm so sorry, Baby."

I had not been able to take care of him and protect him when he needed me the most. I could not do for him what he had always done for me throughout our entire lives together. I always felt so safe, always felt that Thomas would take care of me no matter what. I felt like I had failed him.

"I love you so much, Baby. I'm so sorry."

I tried to sit in the chair next to his bed so I could be beside him all night, but I was so exhausted that I could not get comfortable sitting upright. I stood once more and told him how tired I was, that I could not keep my eyes open, and that I was going to be on the couch in the room, that I was not going anywhere.

"Don't worry. I'm right here with you, Baby."

I knew he could not talk to me, but I knew he could hear me. The nurse brought me a blanket and pillow for my makeshift bed on the couch. I stood over Thomas once more.

"Goodnight, Baby. I love you. I just need a few hours of sleep. You know how I get when I'm exhausted. I just need to sleep for a moment."

I laid my head down on the couch and fell asleep almost immediately.

* * *

I woke up sometime around 5:00 a.m. I was groggy, and it took me a moment to get my bearings. I sat up and looked over at Thomas.

The whistling noise from his oxygen had stopped.

Did he pass already? I thought. *While I was here sleeping and not by his side?*

I laid back down and pulled the covers over my head. I was not ready. I must have lain there for another fifteen minutes before I told myself I *had* to be ready. There was no other choice.

I walked to the reception area and approached the woman at the desk.

"Please, please, please come and check on my husband. I don't know if he's passed away."

She said of course and followed me back to the room. She gently placed two fingers on his neck, then pulled back the covers and did the same at his wrist. Then she turned back to me.

"He's gone," she said.

She marked the time of death as 5:40 a.m. Thomas died within fifteen hours of having arrived at hospice—not the original estimate of twenty-four to thirty-six hours. I would never have taken a nap if I had known that Thomas was going to die while I was sleeping. I was in such agony for not being at his side when he passed away.

Within minutes of his being pronounced dead, two young women came in to clean up the room. They did not even ask me if I wanted some time with Thomas.

"Do you mind if I sit with my husband, please? He just passed."

They agreed, but in a manner that made it seem like I had made some kind of outrageous request. I knew from experience that families sometimes sit with their loved ones for hours after they died, and I felt like even in this, the worst of all possible moments, we still were not getting the respect we deserved. Despite their surprise at my request, the young ladies left the room—only to wait out in the hallway.

I approached Thomas's bed. His face was peaceful. Restful.

"Baby, thank you so much for loving me for forty-five years. You made me such a happy woman. Thank you for always caring about me and tending to my every need. You were always willing to put me first. Please keep loving me and looking out for me, because I still need you, Baby. I know you will. I know you'll always be there for me. I still need you, Baby."

Through tears, I continued to thank him for loving me the way he did, with all the caring and affection he could summon. I took a few more pictures. After about thirty minutes with him, I told the young ladies that they could come back into the room. I gathered my things to leave the room, then stopped in the doorway.

I took one last look back at Thomas, lying there so still. I could not believe that I was leaving him here, that once I walked out that door that my life with the most loving, caring man was over.

I came for a family reunion and left without my family.

With that thought, I walked out the door.

CHAPTER 10

THINKING POSITIVE THOUGHTS

I SAT IN A ROOM RIGHT OFF THE RECEPTION AREA THAT WAS DESIG-nated for family. It was close to six in the morning and too early to call anyone. I knew my sister would still be asleep, as would any of our family and friends out on the West Coast.

So, all alone, I began thinking about Thomas's funeral. We both said we wanted to be buried in California. Both of us considered Los Angeles home.

I did not know how to arrange Thomas's transport to California. The hospice receptionist informed me that in Florida, if a body is going out of state, the receiving mortuary must make all the arrangements by speaking with the mortuary in Florida. With that knowledge, I called Iris Brothers Mortuary in Los Angeles.

The gentleman who answered the phone was clearly not happy to be on call at 3:00 a.m. Pacific time because he was quite short and rude.

I told him that my husband had passed, that I wanted to bring him to Iris Brothers Mortuary, and that we had conducted business with them before.

"Have the mortuary there call us, and we'll be happy to help." He hung up.

Frustrated and irritated, I returned to the reception desk to tell them what he had said. She apologized and said that that was not how they did things in Florida. So, it was back on the phone to Iris Brothers Mortuary.

"I don't care what they said," the man on the other line said. "I'm telling you what you need to do."

At that point, I had had enough. I hung up on him. I'd be damned before I would give them one cent of my money, no matter that my family called on them many times in this time of need. I should have reported him to his supervisor, but it became harder and harder to fight with all I had dealt with in the last couple of weeks.

And that made me angry. I was already so upset about the conditions surrounding Thomas's death and now this, yet another indignity. I decided after the string of indignities, after everything that had gone wrong, that maybe I had some fight left in me after all.

I pulled out my tablet right there in hospice and Googled medical malpractice attorneys. I knew in my heart of hearts that Thomas's physicians had done something wrong. I left messages with three attorneys who were licensed to practice in Florida.

Doing so left me feeling somewhat energized with a new focus. I went back to the reception desk once more and asked her to recommend a Black–owned and operated funeral home for me. She provided me with a list of recommended homes but stated that she was not allowed to advise me about any specific ones, nor was she able to tell me whether or not they were Black-owned.

I was leery of picking any name off the list without knowing who owned the home. Thomas's friend Charles had had a horrific experience with a Florida funeral home when his daughter, Andrea, died while on vacation. The home they used poorly handled Andrea's body, causing it to break down—so much so that they were not able to hold an open casket ceremony in Los Angeles.

I was *not* going to let that happen to Baby.

Still, I did not know who to call for a recommendation. Then I remembered the funeral home in Atlanta and the director who had helped me with my mother's funeral arrangements. I called, left a message, and crossed my fingers.

When he called back, I said, "I don't know if you remember me, Mr. Levy, but you helped me with my mother about three years ago. I don't know if what I'm about to ask will mean any business for you, but I really need your help."

I explained to him the situation I was in—and his reaction was completely opposite to that of the man from Iris Brothers Mortuary.

"Stay by your phone," he said. "I'll be back to you in about thirty minutes."

Sure enough, a half an hour later, my phone rang. Mr. Levy just happened to be attending a conference in South Carolina for Black funeral home directors, and one of his colleagues in attendance owned a funeral home in Orlando. Mr. Levy introduced me to Reverend Porter, the owner of that home, who was also on the call. Reverend Porter took some information from me and told me he would send someone over right away to pick Thomas up.

It was the first sense of relief I had felt in some time—to finally speak to someone who understood that their mission was to care for others and alleviate worry in their time of need.

* * *

At approximately 8:30 a.m., I finally called my sister to let her know Thomas had passed.

"I had a feeling he had," she said. "I've just been laying here, unable to sleep. Now I know why. Did you tell Nichelle yet?"

"No," I said. "Not yet."

"Why don't I go over to her room and tell her? She won't handle a phone call well. She needs to hear it face-to-face."

I agreed.

Later that morning, the three of us met with a counselor at the hospice facility. We were shown to a private room and were asked to start from the beginning—why we were in Florida, what had happened to Thomas, and what we were going to do now that he had passed.

Though I knew the counselor's heart was in the right place, I did not say much. Nichelle spoke the most, and it was good to let her get out what she was feeling.

When our time was up, the counselor told us that her services would be available to us for a year. We thanked her for her time, and we waited in the family area for Reverend Porter's staff to pick up Thomas.

Reverend Porter stayed true to his word. By 9:30 a.m., his team arrived to take Thomas to the funeral home. Meanwhile, the law offices with whom I had left messages started returning my calls. I related my story to them and told them I was considering suing.

Two of the three attorneys I spoke to advised me to get an autopsy— that having one would be critical if I wanted to go to court. Yet the third attorney told me an autopsy would be a waste of my money. If Thomas was in good health before his time in the hospital, all we needed were the records from Everett that demonstrated that.

I did not know what to do. Did I really want to get an autopsy on Thomas? Did I want his body mutilated so I could sue? I thought about researching exactly what happens during an autopsy, but I was afraid to know. *If I don't sue, then I may never know what caused Thomas's death and lose the opportunity to hold those doctors accountable.*

Funny as it sounds, I thought about the legal dramas I had watched on television, where they say if you really want to know what is going on, you should get your own independent autopsy. I had not *actually* decided to file a lawsuit at that point. I had made those calls in desperation, but after considering it further, it made sense to play it safe rather than be sorry later. In my heart, I knew that something had gone terribly wrong with Thomas's care at that hospital. I even believed that there might have been a cover-up so the facts would never be known. Could I walk away and allow those doctors to get away with that? How many families had been affected or would be affected by the actions of those doctors? I decided to get the autopsy.

But the Reverend's team had already left with Thomas's body.

I called him in a panic. "Where is my husband? I don't want you to touch him, Reverend Porter!"

Thankfully, Reverend Porter was cool and calm.

"Everything is alright, dear," he said. "He's refrigerated now, and we were waiting to do anything else until we talked to you." *Of course he wouldn't do anything until I paid him and signed papers giving him that authority*, I thought. *There's no need to panic.*

I let out a huge sigh, then told him I was considering an autopsy and to wait to hear from me. He agreed—but things had gone so badly up to this point that even though he had given me no reason for concern up to that moment, I simply did not trust his word.

"I just want to be sure we understand each other, Reverend. You're not going to do *anything* to my husband at this time. Is that correct?"

"Yes, Mrs. Brown. I understand that we're not to do anything until we hear from you. In fact, I know of a doctor who can perform the autopsy for you, if you're interested. I've worked with him before, and he's done a terrific job. I can arrange that for you if you'd like."

It turned out that the physician he recommended had also been mentioned by one of the attorneys I spoke to. That was confirmation enough for me that this doctor was reputable. I asked Reverend Porter to make the arrangements, and he did so.

* * *

All throughout the morning, friends and family texted, checking in to see how Thomas was faring. I let them know Thomas had passed, which sent my phone ringing off the hook. I did not have the strength to answer. I knew they were concerned and wanted to be there for me, but I could not bear telling the story over and over again. I texted back and let them know that I would call them when I could.

Many still wanted to send money. My cousin Greg, who is a pastor in Birmingham, and my neighbors, the Neals, all offered to come to Orlando to drive us back home. I was touched beyond measure at the outpouring of support. It is one thing to think people care, but it is another to see that care so selflessly demonstrated. There was no question that many people loved Thomas and me.

While I had lost the love of my life, my independent streak remained intact. I thanked everyone for their offers, but Thomas and I had taken our share of road trips in our time, and the drive to Orlando had actually been quite nice. I asked Tommie if she would mind the drive, and while she said she would not be much help behind the wheel, she was agreeable. I was fine to make stops and take our time, since I had no idea how long the autopsy would take, nor did I know how long it would take to get Thomas shipped to California. The peaceful drive on open roads would be just the thing I needed.

The next morning, my sister and I packed up the car and checked out of the hospitality suite at Viewpark. Nichelle decided to fly back instead of making the drive with us. Before we took to the road, we stopped at the funeral home for a noon appointment. I completed all the paperwork and paid for the funeral home and autopsy services. A copy was made of Thomas's medical records to be given to the autopsy physician for his review. When our business was finished with Reverend Porter, we headed home to Atlanta.

The trip was uneventful. We stopped after approximately three hours to stay overnight in a hotel. We were in no rush, and since it was unlikely we would make the trip in one shot, it made sense to travel nearly halfway. When we reached Atlanta the following day, I rushed to the veterinarian to pick up Abby while my sister waited for me at home. When I pulled into the driveway with Abby, I texted a couple of my neighbors who wanted to know when I returned home.

Gail responded by bringing food for me and my sister. It felt good not to have to think about ordering out that night. The gesture was so kind and reminded me of how she and her husband, Orlando, hosted a small welcome party for us when Thomas and I first moved into the neighborhood twenty-four years before, inviting several neighbors in the cul-de-sac.

"Jonnie, the neighborhood will never be the same without Thomas," Gail said. I told her that I know. Thomas was always the life of the party, and everyone looked forward to being in his presence.

There was comfort in being home again, in familiar surroundings, like my own bed. It actually felt good to be around all of Thomas's favorite things—to sit in his oversized recliner, to be in his kitchen, where he made so many healthy and delicious meals for us. I was not missing Thomas just yet.

I went to bed early, not because I was sleepy but because I wanted to be alone to think about Thomas—to cry and to think about how losing Thomas was going to change my life. For all of my life, for over seventy years, I had never lived alone.

Not only that, but I had never experienced this kind of unexpected loss—and I had difficulty processing it. When I had lost my parents, their decline had been slow and gradual. It was also easier to accept because they were ninety-nine and ninety-seven years old; they had lived full lives. My father even told my sister repeatedly that he was ready to go. Even though those deaths were sad, even though they made me cry, the impact on me was so different from this.

I found myself analyzing the events at Viewpark Hospital like I would troubleshoot system problems on my job: How did this happen? Where should there have been checks and balances? Did any checks and balances fail, and why? What could I have done to achieve a different outcome? Why did this happen to us? What could I do to prevent this from happening again?

People would later tell me, "Don't do that. You did everything you could to get Thomas the care he needed." However, analyzing every moment of Thomas's hospital stay helped to solidify in my mind the shortcomings of that hospital, at least in terms of the inadequacy of protocols, internal controls, coordination, and communication.

Things seemed to occur, or not occur, randomly—without process, preplanning, or consultation with those who had relevant information. Medical personnel refused to take action when it was critical and failed to focus on developing a plan to save Thomas's life. Worse still, the doctors seemed to give up on him very early in Thomas's hospital stay, claiming the outcome was already known. I was certain that Thomas would have lived if he were white, or at least a better effort would have been made to help him. All of these were factors in Thomas's cold symptoms leading to such devastating results.

Over time, I would spend hours rehashing my analysis, and then I would always come back to reality, reminding myself that Thomas was gone and nothing was going to change that fact. Eventually, after reading several self-help books, what helped most was thinking about the blessings in my life that I could still be grateful for, instead of focusing on my loss.

Foremost in my mind were the forty-five wonderful years spent with a man who let me know every day that he loved and cherished me; I felt that Thomas had given me enough love to sustain me for the rest of my life, instilling in me such confidence as a woman. I thought about my excellent health, thanks to the healthy meals my mother and Thomas had fixed for me over the years. He loved caring for me and pampering me, so I became terribly spoiled, but I always knew I could take care of myself, if need be. I would have to make adjustments in my life to do everything on my own, but I also knew that I am very capable. I thought about the beautiful home we had remodeled the year before Thomas's death, including his kitchen, and that I would not have to worry anytime soon about house repairs. I was okay financially, and as long as I was prudent, I would not have to worry about making ends meet. I thought about all the things Thomas and I had shared—what we experienced together and what we had accomplished together in our lifetime. We were such terrific partners in *almost everything.*

Thinking positive thoughts in our peaceful home and in our comfortable bed helped me put one foot in front of the other to deal with this inconceivable emotional pain and agony. I had no choice. I had to go on for Thomas's and my family's sake.

But first I had to send him home.

CHAPTER 11

HOMEGOING AND GOING HOME ALONE

THE MORNING AFTER WE RETURNED TO ATLANTA, I BEGAN WORK- ing on the details of Thomas's funeral. Thomas and I had talked several times about preplanning our funeral arrangements, and we were actu- ally going to address the subject seriously when we returned home from the reunion.

Having planned my mother's and father's funerals, I knew exactly what I needed to do. Top of the list was finding a funeral home in Los Angeles to receive Thomas's remains. I was still upset with the treat- ment I had received from the man at Iris Brothers Mortuary, so I knew I would not do business with them.

When I was still at the hospital, I called both of Thomas's childhood friends that I met the night of our first dinner date. Both Charles and Earl had become pastors, and they were a source of comfort for me when I was the most distraught. At the time of Thomas's death, I cried and pleaded with them to help me.

When I called again, I asked them to jointly officiate Thomas's funeral. The three of them had been friends since Thomas moved from Chicago to Los Angeles as a teenager. They ran the streets together, getting into minor trouble, sneaking into the Hollywood Palladium to see James Brown—all the things that mischievous teenagers did. I admired how they had maintained their friendships throughout the years, and because they had, they agreed to my request. They also recommended a number of funeral homes.

I learned that Reverend Porter would need the name of the funeral home in Los Angeles soon, because once the autopsy was completed, Thomas would be transported to the home I chose. Based on limited information and without being able to visit, I decided on Hollins & Reese Funeral Home, a staple in the Los Angeles African American community for decades.

Thomas had once said that he wanted to be buried at Inglewood Cemetery, which is adjacent to Los Angeles, where both his parents and my parents were laid to rest. It is a huge, beautiful cemetery and a very desirable place to bury loved ones, if such a place can be called such a thing. I had suggested that we consider Riverside National Cemetery instead: Thomas had served his country, and he deserved the honor to be buried there on those incredibly beautiful grounds. It is also free, and with me being the practical accountant, I asked him why should we pay for expensive real estate at Inglewood Cemetery when Riverside was free?

"How often have you visited your mother and father at their grave sites?" I asked. "Maybe our children would come visit our grave site, maybe even our grandchildren will visit us since they know us. But the next generation? They may very well never visit us at all.

"Not only that, but I love the fact that there are celebrations at the national cemetery several times a year on Memorial Day, July 4, and

Veterans Day where American flags are placed on every grave, honoring every military person buried there. The cemeteries will always be impeccably maintained. And the most important thing to me as a genealogist are the governmental genealogical records associated with national cemeteries."

Thomas eventually relented. "Okay. You decide. Just make sure we are together."

"Baby, you don't even have to say that. You know I will be wherever you are." We assumed that I would outlive him because I was six years younger and have a long history of longevity in my family. I promised him that we would be buried together, at Riverside National Cemetery.

* * *

About a week before we left for the reunion in Orlando, as I was busy preparing for the trip, Thomas asked, "Baby, you don't know where I take our clothes to be dry-cleaned, do you? I'm going to pick up some things now. Why don't you take a break and come with me?"

I agreed, thinking it would only take a few minutes and I had not spent a good deal of time with Thomas amid all the reunion planning and the writing of the family history book. I did not think anything odd about him showing me the dry cleaner at the time. But maybe somewhere in his subconscious mind, Thomas knew what was about to happen to him and he wanted me to know where he had a relationship with a dry-cleaning establishment.

I decided I would bury Thomas in his tuxedo, so that meant a trip to his dry cleaner's. When I dropped it off, I asked the gentleman there if he remembered me or my husband, to which he said, "Of course." I told him Thomas had passed suddenly, and the shock showed clearly on his face. I asked him if he could promise to have the tuxedo ready for me the next day. He assured me he would.

The next day when I arrived to pick it up, I handed the gentleman my ticket and debit card. He held up his hand and told me there was no charge. He wanted to provide this service for Thomas for being such a terrific customer over the years. Thomas was like that—he made an impact, big or small, on every life he touched. I tearfully thanked the man for his kindness and went on my way.

I searched Thomas's dresser drawers for his bow tie, cummerbund, suspenders, and all the other items he needed to go with his tux. I became frustrated with searching and decided to buy what Thomas needed. Terry, a friend, worked at a men's store, so I called him and told him the situation. He said not to worry and he would drop the items off at my house that evening. That is exactly what he did—and he refused to accept any money in payment. Terry said it was the least he could do for someone who had been so kind to him.

I then gathered paperwork and scanned documents (such as a copy of Thomas's DD214, the military discharge papers) that I would need to provide to the funeral home so they could arrange burial at Riverside. Other items I needed were family information and pictures for Thomas's funeral program and obituary. My plan was to work on that while on the five-hour flight to Los Angeles.

Once Reverend Porter told me the flight information for Thomas to be transported to Los Angeles, I made reservations for flights for myself and Tommie. Michael and Nichelle made their own travel arrangements for their families and would arrive the day after me.

Reverend Porter then called and informed me he needed an extra day to clean up Thomas's body after the autopsy and prepare him for travel. Perhaps I should have asked why he needed the extra time, but something in me said I did not want to know. Besides, I was sure I had no choice in the matter, so I told him it was fine. I did not google what happens during an autopsy until about three years after Thomas's death.

Once I arrived in Los Angeles, I visited the funeral home I had selected—and I was *not* pleased. The facility was older and in sore need of remodeling. It was not the kind of place where I wanted to have Thomas's service, but I was committed at this point. There was nothing I could do.

Earl met Tommie and me at the funeral home. Much to my surprise, he offered to pay for the funeral. It was so kind and generous of him—in fact, too generous for me to accept. I politely declined, despite his insistence. It soon became clear to me that Earl had interpreted my initial plea for help as a signal of some financial need. I assured him that it was not, but it was yet another example of how Thomas was so highly regarded by those who knew him.

* * *

In order to have the burial the same day as the ceremony, we would have had to schedule an early funeral, giving us time to travel to Riverside for an early afternoon burial. I certainly did not want an early funeral, as I was not a morning person. I also knew how difficult this was going to be for me, so the thought of having time between the funeral and the burial was actually quite comforting. I decided to have the burial the next business day following the funeral.

In the middle of all this planning, I received a return call from Dr. Bernard Armstrong, Thomas's primary physician at Everett. "What happened to Mr. Brown?" he said, with much surprise in his voice. He could not believe Thomas had died because the last time he saw him, Thomas was a healthy man with no indication of a serious problem.

I told him I still did not know—that I had taken Thomas to the hospital with what amounted to cold symptoms and the next thing I knew his kidneys had shut down while the doctors continually told me they did not know what was wrong.

"Did Thomas have kidney disease, Dr. Armstrong?" I asked. Thomas was always very good about telling me what the doctor had told him at his visits, or sharing the visit summary with me, and he had never told me anything about his kidneys. Still, I had the man on the phone, and I was not going to waste this opportunity to ask.

"No," he said. "In fact, Thomas's kidneys were in very good shape."

"What about his diabetes?"

"I didn't even classify him as a diabetic anymore because he had it so well controlled over many years."

I continued to relate our story to Dr. Armstrong, and toward the end of our conversation, he made two important points. First, he said a patient's organs should always be monitored while undergoing any kind of treatment. Second, if a physician does not know what is going on with a patient, he or she has an obligation to transfer that patient to another facility where there is the expertise and equipment to treat that individual properly. My own experience with my father confirmed that, while it was not unusual for patients to run into difficulties with their kidneys while hospitalized, the doctors will normally pull back on their treatments if they see the kidneys are being affected.

I thanked Dr. Armstrong for calling me back and being so clear while sharing the information. He repeated his condolences for my loss. As I hung up, my mind churned with what he had just told me, but I did not have time to think about it at that moment. I returned to the planning of the funeral.

* * *

The viewing the day before the funeral was to be held from 2:00 p.m. to 5:00 p.m., but I was in no hurry to get there. Nichelle texted me when she arrived at the home. I had been worried about the fact that Reverend Porter needed another day for Thomas's preparation, so I asked her, "How does he look?"

"Well...if you look hard, you can see it's Daddy."

I finally arrived at the viewing at around 4:00 p.m. Many family and friends were there, and I felt them watch me as I approached the casket. Thomas looked terrible, not like himself at all.

Was it the autopsy? Was it the travel? Did the hospital treatment make him look like this?

Everyone watched and waited to see my reaction. I looked at him for as long as I was able and then finally turned away.

"I don't know who that is," I said. I just could not acknowledge that Baby was in that casket.

I walked away and said hello to everyone there—high school friends, college friends, and coworkers, along with family. Many had driven and flown long distances to be there for us, including my cousins in Nevada and Georgia, and my friend Nancy and her husband, also from Georgia. Despite my disappointment and despair at Thomas's appearance, being surrounded by so many loved ones made it a little easier to take. I will always be grateful for how much love was shown for us in our darkest hours.

When the funeral ended the following day, on Friday, August 11, many came to me offering their condolences. The repast took place at a local restaurant in a private dining room. I asked everyone to order what-ever they wanted. We all enjoyed the time as best we could. Charles wanted to cover the bill for the repast, but I thanked him and said no, realizing that he, too, believed that my cry for help was a financial one. It was special for our family and friends to be together during this time.

Soon enough, the morning of the burial ceremony on Monday, August 14, arrived, whether I was ready for it or not. After the seventy-five-min-ute ride to the grave site in limousines, we lined up in a staging area. I met with one of the military officers, along with a cemetery employee, and they walked me through the logistics of the ceremony. At precisely the scheduled time, all of the cars in the procession made their way to the pavilion, where the formal ceremony took place.

The ceremony was an incredibly moving experience. An American flag had already been draped over Thomas's coffin for the journey to the cemetery. The military men surrounding him stood tall and moved slowly and deliberately as they removed the flag and folded it for presentation to me. Taps played softly in the background. They pulled and tugged at the corners of the flag, turning it with such precision and care into a taut triangular fold.

Once the folding was complete, an officer slowly came to me and bent down on one knee. He looked me solidly in the eyes.

"On behalf of the President of the United States, the United States Air Force, and a grateful nation, please accept this flag as a symbol of our appreciation for your loved one's honorable and faithful service."

He placed the flag in my hands, and it took everything I had to keep from breaking down and crying. Despite all the challenges we had had getting Thomas to this point, the ceremony was quite beautiful and was a fitting tribute for a man of Thomas's stature.

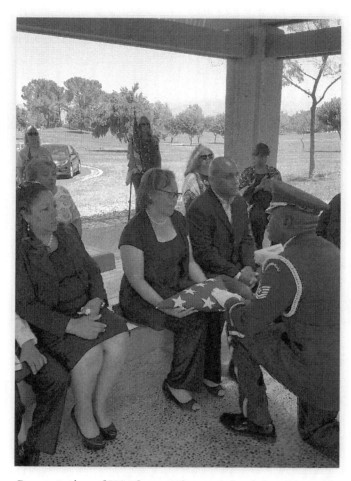

Presentation of US Flag at Thomas's burial at Riverside
National Cemetery. Riverside, CA. August 2017
On front bench: Nichelle, Jonnie, Michael. On second
bench: Tommie, Claynette (sister-in-law), and Mary

* * *

We only had a few moments to stand around and talk, as there were
cars from the next ceremony on their way to the pavilion. We were
not allowed to go to the burial place at that time and would have to

come back at a later date. The limousine took us back to Mary's house, where Tommie and I were staying, and all of us went out to dinner that evening.

After dinner, I told my sister that I was going home with her. I could not bear to go home alone. I called my job and requested a week's vacation. My boss, Doug, was very supportive and could not have been more understanding.

Tommie and I left for Seattle on Wednesday, August 16. When we got to her place, I told her that I planned to sleep late every day, so she was not to worry about waking me in the morning. I was a late sleeper as it was, so it was not too out of the ordinary for me to say such a thing.

During my visit, Tommie and I ate dinner out a few times and watched movies all day. I visited friends that Thomas and I knew while living in the Seattle area, sharing Thomas's funeral program with them all. One of those friends was John and his children and grandchildren. John was the witness at our wedding ceremony, and his daughter Heather had asked Thomas to be her Special Person at school. Sadly, John's wife, Diana, passed unexpectedly about five or six years earlier, so John and I instantly understood each other's grief.

After about five or six days, I told Tommie I had to go home. I had to see about my dog, Abby, and I needed to return to work. I could not avoid that empty house forever, no matter how badly I wanted to.

My neighbors, the Neals, picked me up at the airport, walked me into the house, and told me to look around to make sure I felt safe. After they left, I sat down in my chair in the family room and turned on the television. I looked at the list of recordings on the DVR that Thomas had recorded, most of them cartoons. (Thomas absolutely loved his cartoons—maybe that's why he had such a terrific sense of humor and saw the comedy in everything, no matter what the situation.) Other recordings consisted of his cooking shows and science programs. I began deleting some of the recordings but then looked over at Thomas's empty recliner and began to cry.

I stood, walked over to his recliner, and sat down. I felt like Thomas's arms were around me, and I stopped crying. To this day, I sit in his chair whenever I am in the family room; it is the closest I come to feeling his embrace.

I thought again about my conversation with Thomas's doctor from Everett—and about the calls I had made to the attorneys.

"What happened to you, Baby?" I asked out loud. Then I fell asleep in his chair.

CHAPTER 12

WHAT HAPPENED TO THOMAS

IT WAS DIFFICULT ADJUSTING TO MY NEW LIFE.

When I returned to teleworking near the end of August, I looked forward to logging on to my laptop every day so I could focus on something else. When the workday was done, all I did was think about Thomas and wonder what happened to him at the hospital. I put pictures of Thomas in every room of the house so that, no matter where I was, I could talk to him and see his face. It helped a great deal for me to see and talk to him as if he were there in the house. Still, I kept "running the tape" in my mind about the experience in Orlando. There were just too many troubling and unexplained situations for me to let it go.

Then, sometime in mid-September, I received a call from Dr. Wallace Armstrong, the pathologist who performed the autopsy on Thomas.

Dr. Armstrong wanted to discuss the report that I had received in the mail a few days before, a report I could barely read because all I thought about was how they mutilated Thomas' body to determine the autopsy results. Specifically, the doctor wanted to review with me the general condition of Thomas's organs at death, which were normal, and what he determined to be the cause of his death—gastrointestinal hemorrhaging. He explained that there had been a great deal of blood from bleeding ulcers.

"But Thomas didn't have any ulcers," I told him.

"Ulcers can develop within forty-eight hours," he responded. "The bleed had not been addressed in the hospital."

I sat in stunned silence for a moment. They had done this to Thomas. Whatever they had done to him had not only shut down his kidneys but created ulcers that they did not treat, which caused him to bleed out and die.

"I'm considering suing," I said.

Before I could put a period on the end of that sentence, Dr. Armstrong said, "I would be happy to help you if you want to pursue that avenue."

That was all I needed to hear. Even though I had called attorneys the morning Thomas died, I asked Dr. Armstrong if he could provide references for attorneys in Florida. He gave me three names.

* * *

About the same time that I returned to work, one of the worst hurricane seasons was in progress. Hurricane Harvey in August and September, ranked as the second most costly hurricane to hit the US mainland since 1900, wreaked havoc in Texas and the surrounding areas. Hurricanes Irma and Maria followed a month after Harvey, bringing major damage to Florida, Puerto Rico, and many parts of the Caribbean. Many structures and homes were destroyed, and many people were displaced with no food and basic needs. Power outages occurred everywhere. Senior management at my agency was soliciting every employee who was able to assist the Federal Emergency Management Agency (FEMA) with the aftermath of the devastation. No supervisory approval was required, only a willingness to help.

Wanting to bury myself in something bigger than my personal problems, I agreed to help. In two weeks, I was on a bus to Anniston, Alabama, to the FEMA training center for three days of training. After the training was complete, I found myself on another bus headed to my assigned work location.

Orlando, Florida, of all places.

I could not believe it. I had been hoping for Texas as there might have been an opportunity to visit with Michael and his family. But then I thought, *There must be a reason for this.*

Once in Orlando, I waited for my specific local assignment. With that downtime, I drove to Viewpark Hospital. I sat outside in the parking lot for some time. I even considered going inside to look around so I could remember everything about that place, in case I sued.

But I did not. I knew that nothing good could come of me returning to that place.

It crossed my mind to talk to attorneys while I was in Florida. I knew, however, that once I received my FEMA assignment that I would be working long hours, and when my assignment was over, I would be expected to return to my job immediately to catch up on work. Besides, I was still grieving, and I knew it would be too much for me to take a lawsuit on at that time. I understood full well the time and effort it took to be a part of a lawsuit. I was still trying to figure out how to live my life without Thomas, and I did not want to stretch myself too thin.

It turned out that the assignment to Florida was within one of the most interesting FEMA cadres—Hazard Mitigation—and it was one of the better volunteer assignments. We traveled from county to county every five or six days in our individually rented vehicles, following up with hurricane victims a few weeks after the initial hit to determine their status and provide them with further assistance.

The days were long, and the work was heartbreaking. There were little old ladies crying, living in old trailers that were flooded and now full of mold, yet they lived on $600 in Social Security and had no place else to go to remove themselves from their hazardous environment. There were entire families who had been moved to hotels, but their time was running out, and they had no money to make other housing arrangements. Renters had to contend with landlords who were not repairing the damage to their apartments, because frankly, the landlords were affected as much as everyone else. There were people looking for assistance to replace refrigerators, stoves, water heaters, washers and dryers because they had all been flooded and no longer worked.

One of the most common problems was people looking for assistance with a new roof or roof repair. Sometimes they did not realize there was roof damage until the next heavy rain, ruining their walls, floors, and cabinets. So many of these homeowners did not have insurance to help with their losses. Insurance is difficult to obtain in Florida. Both the rates and deductibles are sky-high due to the propensity for hurricanes, so many homeowners, if their mortgage was paid off, took the risk and declined insurance altogether. Even for those *with* insurance, the policy was often of no help because of high deductibles.

All this to say: this was no vacation. We worked with people in dire straits. Every day, no matter our location, there were long lines of people seeking help. We put in twelve to thirteen hours each day, and I was glad for it. The work left me little time to think about my own troubles.

One evening, I returned to my hotel room and thought, *I have to call Thomas to let him know where I am.* He always wanted to know how I was doing, calling and texting to make sure I was safe. I held the phone in my hand, and when I remembered that he was not there for me to call anymore, I broke down and cried.

Not only was Thomas not there for me to call anymore, but now I had no one who was checking on me once, twice, three times a day like he did to see if I was okay. In spite of all the people who I knew cared about me, I felt so alone. I cried myself to sleep that night—and many nights thereafter. I hurt so much at night.

Those nights in Florida, I repeatedly thought about that autopsy report—about all those specialists who allowed Thomas to bleed to death while under their care. They only thought about their specialty, it seemed, and said nothing about problematic issues that they certainly recognized as doctors. But it was not within the realm of consultation, so Thomas was fine, they said. That thought nagged and nagged at me because those specialty doctors could have raised questions to save Thomas's life. Or maybe they did, and Dr. Chad decided not to address their concerns.

I worked with FEMA for approximately a month and half before returning home at the end of October. The assignment had been exhausting, but I preferred that to being home alone with time on my hands every evening. As soon as I was alone, all I did was think about all the strange things that had happened in that hospital.

For the rest of the year, I spent many evenings with those thoughts. I ran down the list of those events over and over in my head, finally putting them in writing.

I thought about Dr. Zeller, that ICU physician who told me that Thomas was not going to make it and how he would not consult with Thomas's doctor at Everett. How he told me, "No, he's here now," and "I'm not going to have some other doctor running around this hospital." When I reviewed Viewpark's admission packet, I noticed that it specifically stated that hospital staff would be "in contact with your primary care doctor at admission, during your hospitalization and upon discharge. Your hospitalist will partner with your primary care doctor to provide bedside care while you are hospitalized to ensure continuity of care." Why did Dr. Zeller and Dr. Chad not adhere to the hospital's written pledge to patients to initiate contact with Thomas's doctor? Worse yet, why was I told no when I asked for Thomas's primary care doctor to be contacted? The thought in my mind about "property" made me angry, like it was 1860 and Black people had no say over our bodies.

I thought about how Dr. Zeller's behavior was so uncalled for when he told me Thomas was dying. He spoke in such a cruel tone, as though he intended to bring me emotional harm. Why would he talk to me like that? Why would he behave in that manner? He was disinterested in doing everything possible to help Thomas. Had he not vowed to do everything possible to save a life? Where was his moral commitment to the oath he took to become a doctor?

I thought about Thomas's kidneys. His primary physician at Everett said himself that his kidneys should have been monitored and protected when they began their treatments. Why did they not do that? At some point, should they not have realized a problem was developing and stopped what they were doing? Why did they not properly monitor Thomas?

I thought about Thomas's move to the "unofficial" ICU. What the hell was an unofficial ICU anyway? Certainly, something I had never heard of then and have not since. Thomas belonged in ICU *officially*. He was bleeding to death, and it is a known fact that heart attack victims and those who are bleeding are priorities in a hospital. His care was supposed to be so much more attentive there, and yet he did not receive even the most basic level of medical care.

I thought about how Dr. Zeller stood outside Thomas's room, wanting me to see him, and how strange that was. If he wanted to talk to me then, why did he not say something? Why did he not update me on Thomas's condition? After all, he was the one who informed me of Thomas's impending death, and since he was the ICU doctor, he should have been checking on Thomas frequently. Why did he not?

I thought about how Tommie told me she observed that doctors generally seemed to avoid Thomas's room altogether. They would not even look in as they passed. She noticed that Dr. Zeller in particular took the long way around the floor to avoid us after that instance when he stood in front of Thomas's door.

I thought about the span of time where Dr. Chad was off duty for several days. Even though Dr. Hamilton covered Dr. Chad's patients, it appeared that he took little interest in Thomas's condition or how it was developing into a more critical situation. When Dr. Chad returned, he had nothing but condescension for me when I informed him that I wanted Thomas airlifted to Everett, insulting me by asking if I knew that something like that would cost a lot of money.

I thought about the complications with the doctor-to-doctor transfer and Dr. Chad sending me on a wild goose chase; Thomas left alone to lie in his own filth and what the Black contract nurse said about patient care for Blacks in this hospital; the amount of time I was originally told it would take to verify my insurance coverage for the transfer, which was crazy because I was able to determine the coverage in a matter of minutes; the physicians talking to me in jargon I could not understand; the apparent lack of communication in Dr. Chad's care team, seeming never to put their collective heads and knowledge together to come up with a treatment plan to save Thomas's life.

And the blood. The autopsy doctor said there was so much blood. Why did they not treat the bleeding? They knew he was bleeding for some time. Why let time pass until it was a critical situation?

Was it possible Dr. Chad and Dr. Zeller never intended for Thomas to leave that hospital alive? Was it possible that they did something—or *did not* do something—and they would do anything to keep Everett and me from discovering it? They had to be hiding something.

These thoughts consumed my waking moments late into the night, every single night. *We're probably not the first ones to experience something like this in that hospital,* I thought. This happened with too great an ease for this to be an aberration. My thoughts worked me up so much that I knew I had to do something about this.

What happened to Thomas simply could not—and would not—go ignored.

* * *

In early January of 2018, after the holidays, I decided I was going to file a lawsuit.

I discussed my thoughts about a lawsuit with several family members and friends. Some supported me 100 percent. Others questioned my decision and told me I should just move on. "Don't relive the nightmare," they said. I listened to everyone very carefully as their opinions were important to me.

But I listened to *me* most of all.

I knew it would be very difficult to prepare for and sit through a trial, but I also understood that the only way I could ever deal with Thomas's death was for those doctors and that hospital to have to account for their actions. Everyone must know what happened to Thomas and just how horrifying it was for us.

There was never any question in my mind as to what I had to do. "I have to do this for Thomas," I told them. "He has always protected me, and I couldn't help him when he needed me most. I have to get justice for him in some manner, and these doctors should never, ever be allowed to treat another family like this again—especially a Black family."

I contacted the first attorney on Dr. Armstrong's list and explained the situation as best I could with my limited medical background. I thought that, even though I lacked the expertise to explain it from a medical viewpoint, surely a lawyer's interest would be piqued by all of the irregularities that occurred, along with the autopsy and medical records. But I was telling my story to a junior attorney at the firm, and something must have happened in the translation to the decision makers, as I was informed a week later that they were not interested in the case. They did not say why.

I was not deterred. I already knew this was not going to be easy—one phone call was not going to do it. It was a matter of finding the right attorney. So, I moved on. Next.

I saw an ad on television for Ben Crump, the attorney who handled the cases for Trayvon Martin and Breonna Taylor. The ad listed his specialties, one of them being medical malpractice. I wanted Thomas's story to get national attention, and Mr. Crump was a media attorney, so I thought it was worth a try.

Unfortunately, when I called, I was told that my case was not within his specialty after all. Instead, they referred me to the firm of Mathew & Mathew, a firm that was also on the list that Dr. Armstrong provided me. I called them and again spoke to a junior attorney. I then emailed my records.

They, too, were not interested in the case. This second rejection did not faze me, either. I truly believed they had not taken the time to learn what I knew. It seemed that they were looking for the easy case, like when the right leg is amputated rather than the left.

My case was not that type of case, and a focus on detail was required. Truly their loss. Next.

I googled Johnnie Cochran's firm. I had been familiar with them not only because of the O.J. Simpson trial in the early 1990s, but also because of my time living in Los Angeles when Johnny Cochran was the district attorney. I gave them a call, and they sent me a questionnaire to fill out. They also requested the medical records and the autopsy. I wish I could say why I never responded to their requests, but I did not, and after a while, they sent me a letter telling me they were closing the file due to my lack of response. That did not bother me at all.

In the meantime, I found myself gaining confidence as I talked to these firms. I began to understand how they operated and how I could better present my case. I interviewed them as much as they were interviewing me, and in the course of these conversations, I was beginning to understand the kind of attorney that was best suited for me and my case.

* * *

Around this time, I received three separate calls from the Viewpark Hospital collections department regarding an outstanding bill. The first young woman asked for Thomas Brown when she called. *Here is another example of how the people in this hospital do not communicate with one another,* I thought. *They don't even know how Thomas's hospital stay ended.*

I informed the young woman that my husband died while under their care and that she should send the outstanding balance back to the billing department. If billed correctly, they would receive full payment from our insurance.

During the second call from the collections department, I offered up the same response, to no avail. When the manager called me on the third call, I shared the same information, but in her most stern collection voice, she told me that I needed to pay the outstanding balance.

"Are you trying to defraud me? Are you trying to collect money from me over and above the contracted amounts you agreed to accept from Medicare and Blue Cross Blue Shield?" I asked.

The manager's tone changed immediately. "No, ma'am," she said several times.

"Well, listen to me, and listen carefully," I said. "I think you are trying to defraud me. In addition, I believed you killed my husband, so I'm not paying you a dime. If you properly bill the charges, you will get all of your money from insurance. If you have further questions, do not call me again. Put it in writing."

I was offended by those collection telephone calls, but I never heard from the Viewpark collections department again. I assumed that the hospital now knew that a lawsuit was forthcoming.

* * *

Before I ever heard back from Mathew & Mathew and the Cochran firm, I placed a call to Elizabeth Faiella, the third name on Dr. Armstrong's list. She told me I had been smart to get an autopsy and request a copy of the medical records before I left the hospital, as hospitals have been known to alter records. *I like her already*, I thought.

My conversation with Elizabeth was so different from the ones with all the other attorneys. Her firm is a small family-owned firm, so there were no hoops to jump through to speak with her directly. She had been practicing for more than forty years and had only "lost" in court three times, and in those instances, she reached an out-of-court settlement for her clients.

Elizabeth was already interested in my case based on the strength of Dr. Armstrong's referral. She had worked with him before, and she said his willingness to be an expert witness spoke volumes about my case. I liked the fact that she was a woman, and I immediately got a good feeling about her and her politics as we spoke. I felt that if she were to take the case, I would be in good hands.

Elizabeth was different from all the other attorneys in another important way. She went on to explain that she could not tell me at that point whether or not she wanted to take the case because she wanted to consult with some of her expert witnesses for an opinion. I was fine with that, as I also thought it was a good idea to do her research and find out more about Thomas's case before making a decision.

It did not take long.

Each of her experts said my case had merit. One said that Thomas did not even receive *basic* medical care. Another said that medical protocols for what Thomas presented with at various stages were *not* followed. A third expert said that the hospital had *several* opportunities to save Thomas's life but did not. The feeling of validation was almost overwhelming. All those suspicions I had been obsessing over, all those notions that something was wrong in the way Thomas had been treated had now been verified by people who had no special interest in providing anything but an honest opinion, based on the records provided to them.

Elizabeth told me that she only took cases that she could win—cases that would justify the costs to try them in court. I liked that she was straightforward and honest. I liked that she was willing to spend her own money upfront to consult with these medical experts to know the strength of a case. I had a good feeling about her.

Then Elizabeth said something that made me feel even better: she wanted to take my case.

CHAPTER 13

PREPARING OUR CASE AGAINST VIEWPARK

As part of tort reform, the state of Florida has enacted many laws that protect doctors and hospitals from malpractice lawsuits.

One such law is called the "pre-suit" procedure, and it requires the patient or family, before he or she can sue a doctor or hospital, to send a notice with an affidavit from an expert in the same field, attesting to the fact that the attending physician or hospital was negligent. The doctor or hospital in receipt of the pre-suit notification has ninety days in which to decide whether to ignore or deny the claim. Either party can demand that the patient give up the right to a jury trial and submit the case to a three-person arbitration panel. However, non-economic damages for pain and suffering—which is what I was suing for—are limited to $250,000, if the case is decided by an arbitration panel.

Elizabeth was concerned that in this case, the defendants might offer to arbitrate the case and limit the damages to $250,000. This is a tactic taken by a doctor or hospital when the negligence is indefensible and there are no damages to be claimed for lost wages or medical bills claimed. Although the patient or family can refuse to go to arbitration, the law provides if that happens, then at trial, no matter what the jury may award, the patient's non-economic damages are capped at $350,000. This law is onerous, used to deny patients full compensation when the negligence is so clear as to be indefensible. This law actually gives the doctor or hospital a break, if they cannot figure out a way to defend the lawsuit.

On February 7, Elizabeth told me that I needed to become Thomas's legal and personal representative, as required by the state of Georgia. Gail, my neighbor who brought food when I arrived home from Florida, is an attorney, so she assisted me with that legal process. It took about three weeks to obtain the Letters Testamentary document from the Probate Court in my county. When I forwarded it to Elizabeth, she filed the pre-suit.

The pre-suit was filed on March 25, 2018, and Elizabeth held her breath until the ninety days expired—and was both pleased and surprised that no demand to arbitrate the case was made. So, Elizabeth filed the formal complaint in the Ninth Judicial Circuit Court for Orange County, Florida on June 29, 2018. The court date was set for nearly a year and a half later on Wednesday, November 13, 2019.

Meanwhile, I had access to Thomas's medical records at Everett through their patient portal—all his lab work, medications, and summaries of every office visit. When I showed Elizabeth some of the records I had downloaded from the portal, she said, "More." She wanted every bit of information I could find. I downloaded every available document or piece of information and did so quickly, as I was not sure how much longer I would have access to the portal.

However, one visit summary was missing from Everett's records. As I mulled over Thomas's visit summaries, I noticed the one for his July 6, 2017 appointment was missing. This was the day he received a prescription for Bactrim for his urinary tract infection, according to the prescription bottle. The missing summary baffled me.

I sent a picture of his medication bottle to Elizabeth, informing her that the only place he would have received that prescription from was Everett, despite the missing visit summary. She thanked me for it, and I agreed to track down that summary. Elizabeth also requested that I sign a generic medical authorization form that allowed her to officially obtain records from Everett, and any other medical care provider that might be necessary later.

The first week in February, Elizabeth asked that I email her the name of the hospice to which Thomas was transported. She also wanted pictures of Thomas and me. I sent her several, including some of Thomas in the hospital, in the hospice transport vehicle, the nurse checking him to see if he had passed, the flag presentation at Riverside National Cemetery, and his grave site.

In late March, I discovered what happened to Thomas's missing visit summary record from July 6. He had gone to Everett for his urinary tract infection, but they were busy, so Thomas was referred to a nearby urgent care facility. It was there that he was prescribed Bactrim.

I had been so busy with the planning of the reunion that I neglected to look at the visit summary when he got home. He was supposed to have followed up with his Primary Care physician in three days—which he did not do. It upset me to realize I was not paying attention to make sure Thomas followed up with his doctor. I always stayed on top of Thomas's health and his medical appointments.

* * *

The next twenty months were spent in and out of Elizabeth's office in Winter Park, just north of Orlando. In a beautiful, yellow two-story stucco building with a charming courtyard, fountain, and wrought-iron gates, I met her son Peter and daughter-in-law Becki, who make up the rest of the legal team. Elizabeth's support staff—Janice, Jill, and Amanda—are all very dedicated to her and have been with her for a number of years.

It was obvious that Elizabeth had built a competent, cohesive team that worked very well together. Everyone was very welcoming and made me feel comfortable being in their presence, which was a relief as we began gathering documents and having discussions to prepare for the trial.

I had no idea of the volume of information that would be requested from me. Thankfully, as an accountant, I had maintained organized paper or electronic files for most of the requests or I knew how to get the information from elsewhere, if need be.

The opposing counsel requested copies of Thomas's and my birth certificates and our marriage license, as well as our prior marriage and divorce records. I had to provide a record of all of the expenses related to Thomas's funeral. I was also required to divulge my expenses for my time spent in Florida and Los Angeles for Thomas's hospitalization and burial. I provided copies of insurance policies I had on Thomas, a copy of his will, durable power of attorney, and living will or advanced healthcare directive. They also wanted a summary financial statement of all of the assets that Thomas owned and a completed Schedule of Loss of Household Services Information.

I provided documentation from the Veterans Administration that Thomas's prostate cancer was service-related—specifically, exposure to Agent Orange during the Vietnam War—to support his VA disability award. I then had to show evidence of my monthly spousal award from the Veterans Administration. Also requested were Social Security Benefit Amount statements for the last two years for both Thomas and me, current Social Security statements that listed our lifelong earnings records, our joint federal income taxes filed for the years 2012 through 2017, and Georgia tax returns for 2016 and 2017.

All of this was necessary in order to quantify the loss of my husband— as if losing Thomas was quantifiable.

Elizabeth asked me to sign medical representative authorizations relating to Social Security and Medicare. She wanted my cell phone records to see all of the calls I had made to confirm exactly when I made them, which she entered on a timetable. She wanted the completed paperwork for the air transport company that was going to airlift Thomas to Everett.

Elizabeth also wanted a copy of the authorization that I signed for Viewpark Hospital to obtain Thomas's medical records from Everett. When she asked for that, I discovered that I had signed two separate forms. I had completed the second one as an attempted work-around to Dr. Zeller when he refused to call Thomas's doctor for additional health information. I had given the second form to a nurse, hoping she would forward it to the appropriate people in the hospital to request Thomas's records.

I hoped Elizabeth would do more with the document than the nurse evidently did.

* * *

On May 21, 2018, I was scheduled to give an in-person unsworn state-ment in Orlando. I asked Elizabeth if I would be making *just* a statement or if the opposing counsel would ask me questions. She told me that they would ask questions, but that I had nothing to worry about.

As promised, the questions for my unsworn statement were fairly simple. What was my name, and my husband's name? Was I the legal representative for Thomas James Brown? What time period was I in Florida? When did I take Thomas to the hospital? When did he die, and what was my opinion of what was wrong with him? (I used the information from the autopsy to answer this last question.) Was I, in fact, the one bringing the lawsuit? Meeting the defense counsel for the first time and answering these simple questions helped me to get a feel for what the trial might be like, though I knew the actual trial would be a much more difficult ordeal.

It seemed that requests for information kept coming in the months that followed the sworn statement. I signed an authorization to disclose information from BCBS, including billing records. Elizabeth asked for the names and phone numbers of Tommie and Nichelle, as well as others who might possibly serve as my character witnesses.

Elizabeth requested transcripts of all my text messages from the time leading up to the family reunion through Thomas's burial, since I had communicated with many people that way during that time frame. In fact, I deliberately intended for my text messages to document what was going on because I really did not have time to make separate notes at the time. Elizabeth originally asked for screen prints of my texts, but that was almost impossible to do, considering the number of texts. I discovered an app, however, that downloaded texts from my phone and put them in separate PDF files for each person, with date and time stamps for each individual message, making the review of messages very simple.

Elizabeth would often ask me to write about a subject so I could get clarity on it. For example, she asked me to write down the dates and details about Thomas's illness and what finally convinced me to take him to urgent care and eventually the hospital on Saturday, July 22. Elizabeth asked me all kinds of questions about that decision, as it would most certainly come up in court. She also instructed me to write down my complete conversation with Dr. Zeller when he so cruelly told me that Thomas was going to die. These exercises helped both of us to fully understand the situations and to be on the same page as to exactly what happened.

Elizabeth also wanted to know more details about Thomas being diagnosed with diabetes in 1995 and how he managed his condition. As she began receiving the official medical records from Viewpark Hospital, she would email me various notes and ask me to provide further explanations.

At first, I was confused about some of what I read because the notes seemed to be unclear or reflect something other than what had actually happened. It did not take long for me to figure out that these notes were written in such a way as to twist the truth just enough to work on their behalf.

For example, Elizabeth had highlighted in yellow a note from August 1, 2017 indicating that the Case Manager had spoken "to the Patient's wife. The Patient has significantly declined, and she has decided to stop the transfer to Everett and place her husband in hospice."

"No," I told Elizabeth. "That's not correct. Dr. Chad told me that Thomas's organs were shutting down and we needed to make him comfortable. *He recommended* that Thomas go to hospice. I *agreed* to his recommendation. And I didn't stop the transfer to Everett. We were still waiting on word from Everett about the availability of an ICU bed, so the transfer wasn't able to occur. It was still hanging in the balance. I later asked the discharge nurse to cancel the *transportation request,* but only because there was a cancellation clause in the contract, and I didn't want the aircraft to be tied up and unavailable to others. But Everett didn't know that. And I never communicated with Everett after that initial call I made to effect Thomas's transfer to Everett. Any communication with Everett afterwards was a doctor-to-doctor conversation or an update on the availability of an ICU room, as far as I know."

The note stating that *I decided* to send Thomas to hospice troubled me.

"Elizabeth, can *I* decide to send my husband to hospice? In other words, a spouse, even one without medical knowledge, can say to a doctor at any time, send my husband to hospice? And that person gets sent to hospice? That doesn't even make sense to me."

"No, dear," Elizabeth said. "It doesn't make sense. You don't have the authority to send someone to hospice. I wanted you to be aware of the note made in the medical records, and I wanted to hear your response to it. A question will probably come up at the trial."

I was stunned. The doctors and/or the hospital administration were trying to place as much of the responsibility for decisions on me as they could. They were already planting seeds of doubt, even as Thomas was dying.

Or—if what Elizabeth said was true about hospital records sometimes being altered—perhaps after his death.

* * *

I received notice that my deposition would be scheduled for October 15, 2018 in Elizabeth's office, a year before the court date. As the day approached, Elizabeth and I had more frequent conversations to prepare for it.

"I want to give you some guidance," she said, "about what you should wear to this deposition, because you're going to be videotaped. I need you to be a professional, but not too powerful. Don't wear a power outfit. I want you to wear a dress rather than a suit or a blazer. I want you to be vulnerable, got it? A white blouse with a skirt or a simple black or navy dress with a jeweled necklace and simple, not frilly, earrings."

I asked Elizabeth if I could have a picture of Thomas in front of me during the deposition. I just wanted to be able to look at him in case I needed to. Seeing his face gave me strength, and it was a reminder that no matter how difficult this deposition may be, I was doing this to achieve justice for him. Elizabeth and the opposing counsel said that was fine.

The deposition lasted nearly three hours and was challenging. I was first asked specific questions about how we met, where we lived, where we worked, our children, prior marriages, why we were in Orlando, and why I brought Thomas to the hospital. Then many questions followed about the hospital stay, the doctors and other hospital personnel, the Everett transfer, hospice, the funeral, volunteering for FEMA, and other things I did after Thomas's death.

I was doing just fine until I was asked how the loss of my husband had affected me. When I looked at Thomas's picture, I could not keep it together any longer.

* * *

After my deposition, the requests for more information continued. Elizabeth asked for several more documents and pictures. She wanted my updated resume, more pictures of Thomas, and photos of Michael throughout his track career, from junior high school to the Olympics and his professional track career. She wanted pictures of Thomas at those track meets, as well as pictures of me working with FEMA soon after Thomas had passed.

Elizabeth also wanted to see the photo book I created for our grand-kids for Christmas 2018, entitled "Remembering Grandpa." It included pictures of Thomas throughout his life, from the handsome three-year-old little boy with the troubadour haircut combed to one side all the way to the presentation of the folded American Flag to me at the national cemetery. I vowed that as long as I am alive, I will see to it that our grandkids never forget their Grandpa.

Elizabeth's requests for information never seemed to end. She wanted to see Thomas's funeral program; a transcript of my remarks at the funeral (I already had a transcript. I could not speak at Thomas's funeral because I knew I would break down, so I asked Marna to read it for me); my receipt from the hospitality suite at the hospital and the exact days of my stay; a list of all our grandchildren and their birth-days; and Thomas's check-in history at the gym, in case the defense tried to establish that he was some old, frail person, instead of the vibrant, healthy man he was. He was on that weight loss and nutri-tional program—which had helped him lose twenty-five pounds during the last five months of his life—and he had gone to the gym three times a week ever since his cancer diagnosis in 2011. Thomas's doctor told him that the radiation treatments would make him weak, so in order for him to regain and maintain his strength, he exercised for at least forty-five minutes on a regular basis.

Elizabeth also requested the link to my family reunion website. It contained information and pictures from the 2015 reunion in Atlanta and all of the marketing materials for the 2017 family reunion in Orlando. Elizabeth requested pictures of the 2015 reunion with Thomas in them and a copy of all marketing materials for the 2017 reunion. I had planned to update the site after the 2017 reunion with pictures, but I could not bring myself to look at anything related to that Orlando family reunion. Not even today.

Finally, Elizabeth asked me to write out a description of mine and Thomas's plans for the future. She wanted a clear picture of what we were going to do after I retired. That certainly was one of the most difficult things for me to do—to see our plans on paper that would never come to be.

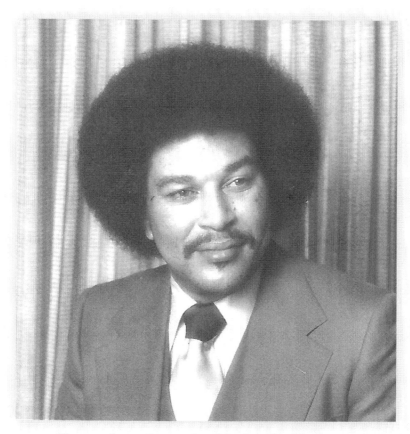

Thomas James Brown. Los Angeles, CA. About 1975

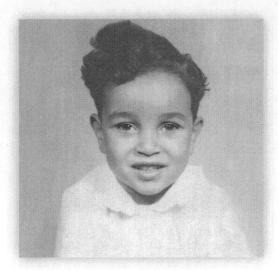

Thomas. Chicago, IL. December 1945.
About three years old.

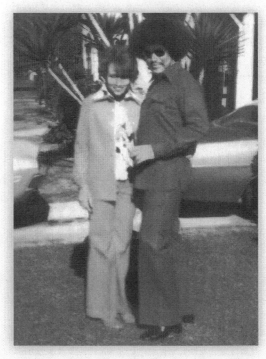

Jonnie & Thomas. Los Angeles, CA. 1970s

CHAPTER 14

I NEED YOU TO BE THE VICTIM YOU ARE

MEDIATION IS REQUIRED IN EVERY CIVIL CASE IN THE STATE OF Florida. The Court requires that the parties in a personal injury case that is in litigation meet in conference in order to try to settle the case before trial. The date for mediation for my case was September 16, 2019 in Maitland, Florida, approximately two months prior to the court trial.

I was pleased that Michael joined me in Florida for the mediation, although the meeting ended fairly quickly. Both counsels were present, as well as the mediator. Both sides presented a mini version of the case. Elizabeth proposed a figure where she wanted to begin negotiations. Then the defense team went to a separate room to consider the offer. The mediator returned alone to our room, stating that the defense did not have the authority to consider an amount of settlement above a certain number, so the negotiations pretty much ended before they began.

So, we remained on course for trial on Wednesday, November 13, 2019.

But something did not make sense to me. We had a great case. *Why didn't the defense request arbitration during the pre-suit period when the damages could not exceed $250,000?* Elizabeth and I would have been terribly displeased with that number, but minimizing the amount of the damages would have been the smart thing for the defense to do. Did they know something we did not know?

Elizabeth assured me not to worry. The defense strategy was to try to wear me down so we would eventually settle for a relatively small amount.

"Elizabeth," I said. "I'm sure you know this already, but I would like to say it again. There is nothing that is going to make me give up on Thomas. I don't care what I have to endure—I am not giving up until I get the justice that Thomas deserves."

* * *

Tommie and my long-time friend Martha gave their depositions in Atlanta to Elizabeth, shortly after the mediation meeting and prior to the trial scheduled for November 13, 2019. Michael and Marna did the same, albeit their depositions were given in Houston to Elizabeth's son, Peter. All of the witnesses answered questions about Thomas and my relationship, our ordeal while Thomas was in the hospital, and how I was coping with my new life circumstances. Elizabeth did not seem to worry that anything said could be seized upon by the defense to work in our disfavor during the trial.

However, Elizabeth did not tell me until a few days before trial about the motions in limine filed by the defense. I was shocked when I heard about the tricks the defense was trying to pull to weaken our case.

Motions in limine are requests made to the judge that certain testimony be excluded from the trial. The defense filed three actions with the court, one in August 2019 and two in October 2019, for the purpose of getting the judge to rule in advance on evidence thought to be prejudicial to the defendant, if heard at trial.

There were about thirty-five motions in limine—attempts to damage our case by making certain evidence inadmissible. As a layman, I could not begin to understand how requests like these to the judge to consider are even allowed. We would not have much of a case if the judge ruled in favor of the defense. Some of the motions in limine were:

The defense did not want us to talk about the failure to effectuate the transfer to Everett. We could not say that Dr. Chad would not call Everett to arrange the doctor-to-doctor transfer, how he delayed doing so, and how he told me it was my responsibility to call.

My sister had testified in her deposition a few months prior to the trial that a nurse at the hospital told her that if it was her husband in Thomas's situation that she would have moved him out of Viewpark right away. The defense claimed this was hearsay information and wanted it excluded. The nurse that my sister was referring to was actually Frances, the same Black contract nurse who cleaned Thomas up on that Sunday, July 30.

The defense did not want Elizabeth to discuss the way Thomas took care of me—how he catered to me and pampered me as a wife, how he pumped my gas and bought our groceries and all the things he did for me as his wife.

They did not want any discussion about Thomas not wanting the feeding tube and that he had pulled it out as a result. The defense claimed this, too, was hearsay and there was no evidence in the record that he did not want the feeding tube.

The defense did not want me to say that Thomas was Michael's father and that he raised him, because he was not his son legally and therefore had no claim in this case. Thomas had not adopted Michael and I had not adopted Nichelle, and the defense found this relevant enough to be excluded. I noted that this was another example of how stepparent relationships are diminished within our culture.

The defense did not want the facts to come out that I had a cybersecurity credential, worked at the Department of Homeland Security, and was one of the first female air traffic controllers at age twenty-three. They claimed there was no factual support for either of these details and that they were therefore irrelevant.

The defense did not want Elizabeth to say that I was trying to save Thomas's life while he was in the hospital.

The defense did not want Elizabeth to raise questions about the hospital's policy and procedure regarding platelets, the amount required for surgery, and how the hospital makes the decision to administer them.

The defense did not want Elizabeth to ask why Dr. Chad did not administer platelets in the opening statement because that was an Argument.

They did not want Elizabeth to ask why the bleeding was not stopped in the opening statement because that was an Argument.

They did not want Elizabeth to ask why Thomas was not formally moved to ICU, if he was so sick, so that he could receive the necessary level of care required for bleeding.

The defense did not want Elizabeth to ask how Dr. Chad had convinced me to give up on Thomas. When a doctor recommends hospice, the notion warrants an in-depth discussion with the patient's family—not the approximate five minutes Dr. Chad afforded me. We never even sat down. There was little discussion. The defense wanted none of that to be included.

They did not want Elizabeth to bring up the note she found in the hospital records that showed Dr. Chad had a pulmonary consult scheduled for Thomas the morning he told me Thomas should be sent to hospice. They did not want her to share that I was never told about that consult.

The defense did not want chart entries from the nurses discussed because they did not affect his care and would only "confuse the jury."

They did not want Elizabeth to bring up the fact that Dr. Chad said if Thomas was going to live, he would need lots of care.

They did not want Elizabeth to use the phrase "abandonment of the patient," indicating that Thomas did not get the care he needed.

They did not want Elizabeth to say that Thomas had suffered a slow and painful death.

The defense did not want Elizabeth to say that Dr. Chad was the captain of the ship in terms of evaluating all the information from the specialists and deciding on next treatment steps.

They did not want Elizabeth to bring up that Thomas had served his country in Vietnam and was exposed to Agent Orange, which led to his peripheral vascular disease.

They did not want Elizabeth to bring up that Michael was an Olympian with multiple Olympic medals, representing his country around the world.

They did not want Elizabeth to state that 90 percent of all children have RSV by age two and that when adults get it, it is a sign for hospitalization, but they seldom die from it.

The defense did not want Dr. Chad's social schedules or vacation days during Thomas's hospitalization discussed.

They did not want Elizabeth to discuss the fact that Dr. Chad did not keep his medical school textbooks, or that he did not subscribe to any medical journals.

They did not want Elizabeth to discuss Thomas's exercise regimen or gym records, that he biked two or three times a week, did push-ups, or exercised thirty to sixty minutes at a time.

They did not want Elizabeth to discuss my conversation with Thomas's Primary Care doctor at Everett after Thomas had passed, when Dr. Bernard Armstrong said that Thomas's organs should have been monitored during treatment and Thomas should have been transferred to a bigger medical facility if the doctors did not know how to properly treat him.

It was hard to believe that motions like these could even come before the court and be considered worthy of a judge's time. The motions concerning my family were particularly troubling and demoralizing to me.

To be frank, I was pissed off. I considered our family to be a unique one. We are all model citizens, pay taxes, and perform our civic duty to vote. Thomas put his life on the line during the Vietnam War as an airman in the United States Air Force—serving his country and wishing he had done more. He had suffered through serious medical conditions as a result of his service, including cancer. Michael wore the United States team uniform with honor and proudly waved the United States flag on foreign land when taking his victory laps around the track. I was a civil servant with a secret clearance—that, in and of itself, was indicative of the extensive background check I passed and the good character I was deemed to have. I was employed by a federal agency whose mission is to protect our country and all of our citizens.

None of this mattered to the defense. Respect, decency, and honor were not character traits they lived by. They were ruthless and heartless, reveling in their legal game of power, money, and expensive suits. Representing doctors and a hospital that allowed my husband to die was acceptable to them, even though these doctors had caused us great harm. But they saw no honor in admitting that. To diminish us was what they must do to make the jury believe something contrary about us. The stakes were high for the defense and their client, so for both of them, any shady maneuver to achieve a win was fair game.

Although I did not previously have strong opinions about the legal profession, I now fully understood why attorneys have such poor reputations.

But all of those motions in limine were allowed to be brought before the court for consideration.

And thank goodness, the judge ruled in our favor on *every single one of them*.

* * *

Just prior to the trial date, Elizabeth told me that when on the stand, she wanted me to talk about my relationship with Thomas, how we met and how we lovingly called each other "Baby." She also wanted me

to write down ten adjectives that I could use to describe Thomas and
our relationship.

"Only ten?" I asked, smiling. I told Elizabeth I would try to narrow it
down—and here is what I wrote, a total of fifteen:

1. Gentle

2. Loving

3. Lovable

4. Charming

5. Sweet

6. Warmhearted

7. Attentive

8. Respectful

9. Playful

10. Loyal

11. Handsome

12. Sexy

13. Wise

14. Giving

15. Irreplaceable

I emailed Elizabeth the list, along with additional comments. I wrote that I often told Thomas that he was a gentleman and a gentle man. He was so kind to me and made me feel so very special. I felt like the luckiest woman in the world because he loved me so much and showed me that love every day.

Despite Elizabeth's preparation efforts, however, there was an issue that nagged at me for months. I mentioned to Elizabeth on several occasions that it was clear the hospital did not give Thomas the best of care and they were trying to hide that fact. I believed that their goal was to never let Thomas leave that hospital alive. I felt with all my heart that what happened in that hospital was a cover-up.

Each time I raised this issue with Elizabeth, she would shut me down and tell me not to say that. After about the fourth time of her telling me that, I asked why. If I understood why, then I wouldn't keep thinking along those lines and making those statements. She explained that those types of assertions were of a criminal nature and that this was a civil case. If I were to say those things in civil court, the judge would throw out the case. We could point out all of the things they did wrong or what they failed to do, but in civil court, we could not accuse them of a criminal act.

"Oh, now I understand," I said. "That's the explanation I needed to hear."

"Let's get this civil action out of the way, and then we can deal with the criminal action. I'm so sorry this happened to you and Thomas," Elizabeth added.

"Elizabeth, you don't need to apologize. You're confirming for me what I think I've known all along."

"There's something else you need to know, dear," Elizabeth said. I steeled myself for what would certainly be more bad news. "Thomas was sent to hospice prematurely. He was actually getting better on his own. They weren't treating him. They gave him fluids and pain meds, but they weren't *treating* him. That's how healthy he was. If they had waited on the pulmonary consult, they would have discovered the issue that required him to be on supplemental oxygen and they could have fixed it. If they had given him platelets, they could have performed the surgery. There would have been no need to send him to hospice."

Thomas could have lived.

I broke down. How much more was there to this horrific nightmare? Thomas could not speak at the time, but did he know what was happening? Did he think that he could live, if given the chance? Was he silently pleading with me to save him? I could not handle this anymore. I was at the end of my rope. It took me a while before I was able to listen to what Elizabeth wanted to tell me next.

"You're emotional right now, Jonnie, and you should be—but I want you to remember something. I know you've had to fight all your life because you're a woman. And I know you've had to fight all your life because you're a *Black* woman. But I need you to be vulnerable when you're up on that stand. I need you to be the victim that you are. I need the jury to see you that way. I don't want them to see you as a strong Black woman, even though you are that. I want them to see you as the victim, because you are that too."

Never in my life have I taken on the victim role. I have been a victim countless times, but I never had the victim mentality. So, in many ways, it was a hard concept to even consider. I instinctively fight to protect myself when I think it is necessary. Still, I understood her point. If we were going to win, I had to do exactly as she said. I had to be seen as the victim.

Elizabeth gave me further instructions. No matter what is going on in the courtroom and no matter what is being said, I must show no emotion and I must be expressionless.

We had an excellent case. Elizabeth was confident we were going to win.

I just hoped, when under further duress, I could do what she asked me to do.

* * *

I had trouble dealing with the premature hospice decision. I wanted to hide or to sleep so I could not think about it anymore. I needed an escape. My emotions were always on the surface, causing me to break down over almost anything.

I found myself constantly thinking about what I could have done to make a difference in the outcome of Thomas's situation—a useless exercise, I know, but that is what happens when a tragedy is so hard to accept. In an odd way, I think it helped me for a while because it gave me something else to focus on rather than the tragedy itself. Yet, it was a waste of time because, bottom line, Thomas was gone and there was no way I could change that.

If I had not sued, I never would have known the truth about the cause of Thomas's death. Regardless of how painful it was, I wanted to know everything that occurred in that hospital.

CHAPTER 15

INSULT TO INJURY

THE TRIAL DATE—WEDNESDAY, NOVEMBER 13—FINALLY ARRIVED.

The day before the start of the trial, I flew into Orlando, as did Tommie coming from Seattle. Michael and Marna planned to come to town on the night before their respective testimonies in court, and my friend Martha was already in town visiting a friend.

Tommie, Martha, and I stayed together in a hotel suite I reserved close to the courthouse. Because Tommie and Martha could not be in the courtroom until after their testimony, either Janice or Amanda from Elizabeth's staff would pick me up every morning and drop me back off at the hotel after court.

Elizabeth had asked the Court for eight days on the court calendar, including jury selection time. On the first day of jury selection, the judge warned that there would be no opportunities to extend the number of days for the trial, as she was assigned to another case on Monday, November 25. It was a warning she would continue to issue, and it kept everyone on edge throughout the trial.

I was already nervous because a new judge had been assigned to our case at the last minute. The defense saw this as an opportunity to bring up those motions in limine again. I knew these high-powered corporate attorneys would continue to try anything to win.

Thankfully, the new judge was tough and was not having any part of this last-minute maneuvering. She told the defense that the decisions already made on those motions still stood. Regardless, it disgusted me to see the defense try to get over on the judge. I was getting the sense, though, that the defense had more tricks up their sleeve to swing the case in their favor, in spite of the overwhelming strength of our case.

Their attitude of entitlement did not stop there. The rules of the court specified that the defense needed to be seated at their table when they were not speaking. Instead, one of the attorneys walked around the courtroom in thought as though he owned the place. The judge yelled at him to stop walking around her courtroom and to sit where he was told. I had never been in a court trial before, so to see him get his comeuppance in that way was, I will not lie, quite amusing.

* * *

For jury selection, we were asked to turn our chairs so we could face the spectator section of the courtroom, where they had seated forty potential jurors. The judge explained in general terms what the case was about and that the attorneys for both the plaintiff and the defense were going to ask questions of them to aid in their selection. If any of the potential jurors felt they had a conflict of interest or any particular issues that would not allow them to serve for eight days, then they were told to raise their hand right then and state why they should be immediately released.

A few people were immediately released; for the others, these questions were posed:

- Have you ever worked for the hospital in question?

- Were you ever a patient at said hospital?

- Do you have any preconceived notions about this hospital?

- Have you had any experience at any hospital, good or bad, that would influence your opinions?

- Do you work in a healthcare field?

- Have you been a juror before?

- Do you feel you can be objective, listen to both sides, and come to a fair conclusion?

If a juror felt a question pertained to them, they raised a numbered paddle that they had been given. When called upon, they often had to answer even more questions posed by the attorneys on either side, such as:

- What do you do for a living?

- What television and/or radio stations do you tune into for your news?

By the time we approached the end of the day, many jurors had been dismissed for various reasons. Neither Elizabeth nor the defense felt that a suitable jury could be selected from the remaining potential jurors. Time was running short, but Elizabeth said we needed to interview fifteen additional jurors the following morning. She did not want to interview another forty, but she felt an additional fifteen jurors would give us a decent pool to select from.

Fifteen more potential jurors were brought in the next morning, and they went through the same process. Knowing the value of having Black people on the jury, Elizabeth zeroed in on a Black man who was a pastor and seemed like such a nice and fair-minded person. I could hear the kindness in his voice when he responded to the questions. Elizabeth also liked a Black female teacher who was low-key and quiet.

Meanwhile, Peter and Becki were busily documenting all the potential jurors' responses and accessing a service that captures all public information available on the jurors. When it came time to make the actual juror selections, Elizabeth and her team had quite a profile on each one of the potential jurors to help us understand their values and beliefs.

The judge reminded us again of the tight time constraints and that we needed to move quickly.

I learned that "picking" a jury is really a misnomer. The attorneys do not *pick* who they want. Rather, they *strike* jurors they *do not* want.

The order in which the potential jurors are seated is important, but it is randomly decided when they line up before entering the courtroom. When seated in the courtroom, they are placed in four rows of ten persons across. The actual jury would consist of six jurors and one alternate. Theoretically, if no one was struck from the first seven people in the first row, they would comprise the jury, with the seventh one being the alternate. If one of the people in the first seven seats is struck by an attorney, the next person becomes a potential juror. Therefore, it matters quite a lot how people are seated in the rows.

The attorneys for both sides ask their questions to determine which potential jurors would be unsuited for their side of the case. Then, the attorneys have two ways to get rid of a juror: a challenge for cause or a peremptory challenge.

A challenge for cause means that an attorney can show the judge that a juror is biased and therefore should be removed. There were *many* challenges for cause in our case because a number of people expressed sympathy for me. As a result, those people were taken off of the potential jury panel.

The peremptory challenge is a "freebie," and the attorney can use it for any reason. Each side gets only three freebies, but has unlimited challenges for cause.

Elizabeth was pleased to see that there were two Black potential jurors within the first two rows and three more potential Black jurors were seated on the back row at the far end of the seating chart. While the Black pastor and teacher were being questioned, both of them were attentive and did not express any bias that would prevent them from being seated. Several other potential jurors had experienced negative treatment from doctors or hospitals, including Number Three, a white woman my age who had actually filed a malpractice lawsuit—definitely grounds for a challenge for cause.

After many of the challenges for cause were heard and several jurors were removed, it was clear that we had reached both the pastor and teacher; they would probably be on our jury, as long as the defense did not strike them with their "freebies." Elizabeth was thrilled that we might actually have Black jurors sitting on my case because not only were they my peers, but it was—and is—quite rare to get Black jurors on a case in which the fate of a Black plaintiff is to be determined.

The defense attorney objected to both the pastor and teacher using his "freebie" challenge. Elizabeth objected on the basis that the exercise of the peremptory challenge was race-based. This shifted the burden to the defendant to demonstrate to the court that it was *not* a race-based challenge and that there were other supposedly good reasons the defendant's attorney had for the decision to remove the jurors. The defense counsel gave their reasons, and they were satisfactory to the judge. Although Elizabeth disagreed, her objections were overruled.

We lost the pastor and teacher as jurors.

Elizabeth was so disheartened at the overt racism of this tactic. I sought to comfort her but not before asking, "Why are you so surprised?"

I was not surprised at all.

Adding insult to injury, potential juror Number Three was allowed to sit on this jury—despite the fact she had actually sued a physician. Apparently, the defendants were more afraid of seating Black jurors than having a biased juror who had previously filed a malpractice lawsuit.

Yet again disappointing—but not surprising.

After the swearing in, we all took our seats. I silently started crying.

Elizabeth leaned in and whispered, "Are you upset because the Black jurors were dismissed?"

Of course, that was part of it. I was also distressed because these jurors knew nothing about me and Thomas, yet they would be the ones to decide this case. The needless loss of my husband, the loss of my life as I knew it, all my suffering for over two years—six jurors would decide if I was due a legal remedy from this court, and all six jurors must come to a unanimous decision.

Are they smart enough or will they be attentive enough to understand what happened medically? Will they be objective? Will they be fair to me, a Black woman? Do they already favor the defense, either consciously or subconsciously? All of these questions hit me at once while looking at their faces in that jury box, and I just could not hold it together.

But none of my thoughts mattered now. Elizabeth and her team had worked hard to prepare us for this moment.

It was time for the trial to begin.

PART III

THE FIGHT

CHAPTER 16

OUR OPENING ARGUMENTS

AFTER THE JURY SELECTION WAS FINALIZED, WE WERE EXCUSED for lunch. Elizabeth and her legal assistants did so much to make me feel comfortable, bringing lunch, snacks, and drinks so that we never had to leave the courthouse. She and her entire staff always ensured that I was doing okay, all things considered.

After lunch, Elizabeth was scheduled to give her opening argument. She had prepared a PowerPoint presentation, as well as several charts and graphs on poster boards, for visual aids for the jury during her opening argument; additional poster boards were leaning on the jury box wall that would be referred to later in her presentation. The judge asked Elizabeth if she was ready to proceed, and she indicated that she was.

Elizabeth is petite, very attractive, and has a great presence. She is about my age, always dresses professionally, and brings a touch of style and sass to her look. I teased her son Peter at one break during the trial, asking, "How does a young man handle having a mother who is so pretty and captivating?"

He joked, "Shhh, don't tell her," but then seriously commented that that is what makes her so effective and compelling.

Elizabeth had described her life to me in a most interesting way. She says she was born with a "straight flush"—that is, good parents, both of whom were also attorneys; great health; access to money so she has never experienced an unmet financial need; good looks; and love from her children and her current husband, who adores her very much. She says she has a duty to be happy and thus is an adventurer, frequently traveling to Italy and the Bahamas. *Vivi la tua vita* is her motto: live your life.

Elizabeth also conveyed to me that she feels fortunate to be a lawyer and to be able to pick cases that she truly believes in. Most of her clients are older—in their seventies, eighties, and nineties. Other lawyers prefer to not take these cases, but Elizabeth believes that the time left for older clients is precious. Understanding that ageism is prevalent in medicine, Elizabeth believes she can do a good job representing these clients.

* * *

Elizabeth prepared well for our case and almost always spoke from memory. As with almost everyone in the room, I was mesmerized when she spoke. I could not wait to hear her statement.

"Good afternoon, everyone," she began. "We're happy to have you here. I'm going to describe what we believe the evidence will show about a story that occurred over a period of twelve days at Viewpark Hospital in July 2017—a little more than two years ago. Most of the story takes place in the hospital during this part of the trial. I'll be using a few medical records, charts, and other materials in my presentation. Our job as attorneys is to make sure we can translate for you the medical information we will share."

Elizabeth stood by one of the poster boards that was already set up, facing the jury.

"I want to start with the twenty or so words that I call 'alphabet soup,' meaning initials that we will hear over and over again to represent these words. You will need to understand what they are because you will hear them often. But first, I'm going to start with the word 'hospitalist.' Formerly, when a person became a patient at a hospital, their primary care doctor, after being in the office all day, would come and see them when they made their hospital rounds.

"But things have changed now, and many primary care doctors don't go to the hospital anymore. So, a new specialty developed consisting of doctors who only practice in the hospital and serve in the role as a primary care doctor. They are called hospitalists. That's what we're talking about in this case—two hospitalists that provided care at View-park Hospital. Dr. Chad was one of them. The other one is his partner, Dr. Hamilton.

"There is a group of about twenty-five hospitalists who serve the role of primary care doctors in this hospital. Their job includes taking care of patients and coordinating their care until they are discharged. They call in specialists who give recommendations and the hospitalist may or may not accept these recommendations. The hospitalist is in charge of all communications, is the point person, the captain of the ship, the one in charge, and the one who should know what's going on at all times. In this case before you, many specialists were consulted.

"I'd like to give you a general idea of this case. Mr. Brown came into the emergency department on a Saturday morning, July 22, and was admitted into the hospital. He had a cough and a slight fever, and he had lost control of his urine at least once. That is, he had a period of incontinence. So, he was admitted for observation. Dr. Chad was the doctor, with Dr. Hamilton as his partner. These are the only two doctors who we are concerned with in this lawsuit.

"Dr. Chad saw Mr. Brown on Saturday, July 22, Sunday the twenty-third, Monday the twenty-fourth, and Dr. Hamilton saw him on Tuesday, July 25, Wednesday, Thursday, and Friday, July 28. Then Dr. Chad came back for the last five days of Mr. Brown's life. So, these are the hospitalists.

"They consulted with the first specialist, an infectious disease doctor, because Mr. Brown had a fever. Then, as I'll explain in a moment, a kidney specialist was called in, as well as a hematologist who specializes in blood disorders. Another specialist is the gastroenterologist who deals with the stomach.

"All of the specialists were called in for consultations, and they gave recommendations to the two hospitalists. In general, the specialists don't write orders; they give recommendations. There's a lot of protocol in this system and rules to follow. That's the general idea of how hospitalists work with the specialists."

I could see in the jurors' faces that they seemed to be following everything being said so far, and this boosted my confidence in Elizabeth's ability to make them understand.

She continued on, "Now here's my list of words that you will hear a lot, so I will define them for you to help you. These doctor specialists have initials, and the whole words are not said sometimes. ID stands for infectious disease. IMG is an internal medicine group—that's what the hospitalists are called. GI means the stomach guy. You'll hear the word scope, which means they'll put a tube down your stomach with a camera to look for a bleed. This afternoon, one of our witnesses will be a blood specialist, a transfusion medicine specialist from Everett. He will talk to you and teach you more.

"Let's talk about blood, okay? Blood cells, the soldiers that go to fight. When you have an infection or injury, white blood cells rush to the site and, on tests, their count changes. There are also red blood cells that carry oxygen to all organs of the body, and then there are platelets, cells that look like plates. When there's a bleed, the platelets will transform. They change, and they have arms and legs that stick together and form clots. They're really kind of amazing. And we'll talk even more about platelets later. The name of the test for your red blood cells is called a hemoglobin test. It should be at a level of twelve to fifteen or sixteen. We're going to talk a lot about hemoglobin."

Elizabeth had to not only argue our case, but she had to educate the jury to get them up to speed—and she was doing a terrific job of it. Still, I worried. I remembered how much difficulty I had with physicians speaking medical jargon to me and giving me so much information all at one time. With that in mind, I watched the faces of the jurors closely for any indications that Elizabeth's information might be going over their heads—not that there was anything I could have done about it. However, they appeared engaged, which gave me some sense of reassurance.

Elizabeth continued with her opening argument, "There is another test that is very important that is related to your kidneys. Your kidneys take care of the waste in your body. If there is something wrong with them, this thing called creatinine will start to build up and get high—and that's bad.

"Now, a couple of illnesses. We're going to talk about RSV. It's a respiratory virus. This is the bug Mr. Brown was found to have. They swabbed his nose on Tuesday, July 25. Tuesday, July 25 is a big day in this case.

"A few more terms. Afebrile refers to the fact that you *don't* have a fever. So, when infectious disease doctors say afebrile, they mean your temperature is below a hundred. Melena sounds like a beautiful thing, but it's not. It refers to blood in your stool. Black stool is a sign of bleeding in your upper intestine, and you'll hear melena over and over again.

"Another word—colonization—means you have a bug that's not bothering you. In other words, we all have bacteria, good ones and bad ones, and the good ones are referred to as a colonizer. That just means that it's not making you sick—it's just something that comes from being human, and we'll talk more about that. Lastly, AKI means acute kidney injury. It means something injured your kidneys, and you'll see and hear this acronym a lot too."

Elizabeth moved to stand in front of the jury and faced them directly.

"In order to understand this story, I'm going to talk to you about two things that are happening at the same time. One is what's happening during those twelve days while Mr. Brown is a patient in the hospital. The other is what's happening to Mrs. Brown in her head and in her heart during the twelve days she's in that hospital. I need to introduce you to who they are and why they were in Florida, and then we will talk about some of the medical evidence."

Elizabeth frequently looked at me as she went on to tell them about our thirty-eight years of marriage; how we met in California; our previous marriages and our children from those marriages; how we helped each other through college; the degrees we earned and the position I held with the Department of Homeland Security; Thomas's self-employment as a real estate professional; Michael's participation in the Olympics and our family's involvement with the Olympics in the 1980s and 1990s.

It was somewhat uncomfortable to have all these things spoken out loud to so many people we did not know while they looked at me, but I knew it was necessary. Elizabeth did not just want this to be about cold, hard facts. She wanted to make Thomas and me human to this jury—to have them see us as real people, not just plaintiffs in a case.

"Mr. Brown was a healthy seventy-four-year-old man," Elizabeth continued, pacing in front of the jury. "He was a type 2 diabetic and took one pill called Metformin and another pill for diabetes that he was about to be taken off of. He was also on a mild pill for high blood pressure that was well under control. He was very particular about staying on top of his health, and both of the Browns established a nearly twenty-five-year relationship with Everett Hospitals and Clinics in Atlanta. Even when Mrs. Brown worked in Washington, DC, they returned home to Atlanta often and scheduled their doctor appointments with Everett."

Elizabeth paused, appearing to be in thought. When all eyes of the jury were fixed on her, she began again.

"That becomes important here. One of the doctors you will hear from is Dr. Bernard Armstrong, who was Mr. Brown's primary care physician at Everett. Let's clarify. There were two Dr. Armstrongs. One is Mr. Brown's primary care physician at Everett, and there is Dr. Wallace Armstrong in Florida, who performed Mr. Brown's autopsy.

"As we said, Mr. Brown was a type 2 diabetic, and he was particular and aggressive about keeping his diabetes under control. He went to the doctor often and even emailed his doctor whenever he had questions about his health. There were emails in his records where he asked questions about his blood tests, which he got regularly. So, we know exactly what his hemoglobin numbers were in early July right before he came to Florida."

Elizabeth walked close to the table where I sat with Becki to my right and Elizabeth's empty chair on my left. Elizabeth turned around to the jury, hand on her chin, her elbow resting on the other hand. She paused to make sure she had the jury's attention.

"We also know that Mr. Brown had never been treated for kidney disease in his life. He had never been treated for anemia in his life. He had only been in the hospital one day in his life, when his doctors placed stents—tubes that open your arteries—in his legs to increase circulation. And they were effective.

"He took good care of himself. He exercised the Monday before they came to Florida at LA Fitness. We have the gym records. Mr. Brown loved to cook, and he did all the cooking since he was retired, and Mrs. Brown was still working. He had lost twenty-five pounds in the last six months through a weight loss and nutrition program just before he came to Florida. He was very conscientious about his health, as was Mrs. Brown. Now here's the general order of what happened."

Elizabeth walked to the poster board showing the calendar and explained in detail the timeline of our arrival in Orlando. She explained how Thomas did not feel well and did not participate much in the events of the reunion. She then walked the jury through the first time he lost control of his bladder, our trip to urgent care, and their recommendation that he go to the emergency room.

"They went to Viewpark Hospital. The hospital took twenty-five tests, all which came back normal. Normal urinalysis, normal blood hemoglobin, normal creatinine, normal chest X-ray, normal lungs. However, he had a fever of only 99.4 when he first arrived, and quickly thereafter, his fever started to spike."

Elizabeth told the jury that Dr. Chad recommended that Thomas stay overnight in the hospital for observation. She told them how Thomas did not want to stay but that I convinced him because of my concern about his lack of eating and drinking water.

"Mr. Brown was treated by consultants that were brought in by Dr. Chad to find out why he had this fever. Mr. Brown was also given medications while they tried to figure it out. The phrase they use for this is *empirically treating* you. This means it's a medical guess. Empirically means, 'We don't know what you have, but we're going to give you these medications and try to treat this fever,' which was concerning."

Elizabeth walked over to another poster board set up on a second easel.

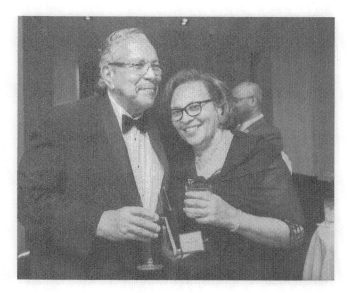

Thomas & Jonnie at a neighbor's wedding.
Atlanta, GA. May 2016

"So, they gave Mr. Brown a series of antibiotics with the assistance of an infectious disease person. Here's a list of the seven antibiotics that Mr. Brown was given and when it was given to him. Recall Mr. Brown has stents to keep his arteries open. He was also on two blood thinners already, which do exactly what they say. One is called Plavix and the other was aspirin. So, he came in with blood thinners on board—and then he was given Heparin, another thinner, to prevent clots, given on top of the two he was already taking.

"Mr. Brown was then given erythromycin—that's an antibiotic. Then Heparin again. Then more aspirin. His Plavix was still in his system. Then Heparin again. Then more erythromycin. And you can see Dr. Chad is prescribing these—not the medicines Mr. Brown came on board with, but the rest of them.

"Then the infectious disease people come, and Rocephin, an antibiotic, is prescribed. Then they switched to one called Amikacin. Then he's given ibuprofen four times, and then he's switched to acetaminophen. Then by day three, Monday, July 24, he gets the last two, ibuprofen and Piperacillin, another antibiotic."

Elizabeth continued to refer to the list of drugs on the poster board.

"Then he was given Omnipaque. That's a contrast material that you take by swallowing so they can take a picture. They did a CT scan of his abdomen to see if they could find out what was wrong with him—why he was having a fever in spite of the treatment, trying to figure out what to do.

"On day four, Tuesday, July 25, a lot was discovered. A lot of things happened. There were side effects. All these drugs they had given him—the ibuprofen, the Omnipaque, and Amikacin—are damaging to the kidneys. The antibiotics which they gave in combination irritated the stomach. And so, you'll hear testimony about the effects of the treatment, of the medicines they were using to treat him.

"Also, on day four, Tuesday, July 25, the mystery was solved as to what the bug was. The nasal swab they took showed RSV, a respiratory virus.

A virus is not treated with antibiotics; it's treated with antiviral medicine. RSV in a healthy adult is kind of a benign disease. As you will hear from the infectious disease experts, it's dangerous in children and people who are ill, people who have cancer, HIV—people who are really sick.

"But generally, it's treated with support like fluids and aspirin. It feels like a cold. A respiratory virus."

That statement caught my attention. *Fluids and aspirin.* That was all Thomas needed? Yet they administered all these other medications that affected his kidneys and stomach. I scanned the faces of the jury again to see if it had registered with them as it had with me. Their faces revealed nothing, although several jurors were taking notes.

"So, once it was discovered what was causing the high temperatures, the antibiotics were stopped because they do nothing for a virus. And the infectious disease people were going to say he was doing well being off the antibiotics. When you look at his temperature, on this chart over here that shows his temperature and heart rate throughout his stay in the hospital, you see the spikes, but by Wednesday, his fever broke and he was never above 100 again. He was considered to be afebrile for the rest of his life. He had cleared the virus.

"Interestingly, when your fever is up, experts will tell you that for every degree your fever goes up, your heart rate goes up ten beats. There's a correlation to it. We will see that Mr. Brown's heart rate got higher and higher and higher, until he cleared the virus, and then dropped back down to a normal heart rate."

Elizabeth walked toward the jury box to make sure the jury refocused their attention on her.

"And then something started making the heart rate climb again. Remember what I told you about your kidneys and creatinine? What we know is that during this period of time, he was getting those medications—Amikacin, which is hard on the kidneys, and the contrast required for the CT scan—both of which were given on Tuesday, July 25. And now we had the kidney injury. The kidney injury was evident on Tuesday, July 25.

"By Friday, July 28, Mr. Brown was placed on dialysis to start washing away waste—and it was working. In other words, he was getting better. He was on dialysis every day while they were restoring him from this kidney injury that was a result of the medication—a kidney injury that he *did not have* before he came to this hospital. The treatment received by the hospital caused the kidney injury."

Elizabeth paced in front of the jury box saying nothing for a few moments, giving the jurors time to make notes. Then she turned to them.

"The other injury Mr. Brown experienced was the irritation to his stomach due to the medicines they gave him. This injury started to make his hemoglobin fall. Recall the hemoglobin measures the red blood cells, which carry oxygen. Mr. Brown came to the hospital with a hemoglobin of eleven. We know his baseline was 11.7. And when I say baseline, it means the last test he had at Everett. The hemoglobin rose from Mr. Brown's baseline of about 11.7, and then it began to drop.

"A one-point drop in hemoglobin, you will learn, is equivalent to about a pint of blood. Mr. Brown's hemoglobin began to drop all the way down to below *seven*. Seven is critical, meaning you have to be transfused. Transfusions were given to try to get his hemoglobin back to normal, but that did not work. In other words, the transfusion should have raised his hemoglobin, but it didn't. Every pint transfused should raise his hemoglobin a point. Mr. Brown got one pint on Friday, prescribed by Dr. Hamilton, and Dr. Chad and Dr. Hamilton gave him two units on Saturday, two units on Sunday, and only one on Monday."

Elizabeth pointed to her charts again. "You can see that the six units did *not* raise his count by six points. They didn't bring his hemoglobin back to where he was when he arrived at the hospital.

"The hematologist was brought in to help figure out what's wrong. Mr. Brown's hemoglobin was dropping and dropping rapidly, so the hematologist ran a lot of tests to detect various blood issues. The tests showed that Mr. Brown had none of the problems that he was tested for. They then tested his bone marrow. Was it not working? They couldn't figure it out for a while."

Elizabeth paused for a moment and then gestured to me. Elizabeth told the jury she wanted to stop and take a moment to talk about our marriage—about how Mr. Brown had been my protector, the one who took care of me, and how our roles had been reversed by this situation. She explained that while I was well educated, competent, and a problem solver, I was very much out of my element when it came to hospitals and medicine.

Elizabeth also pointed out that the doctors did not know what was wrong for some time and were not able to tell me much. She told the jury how difficult that was for me.

"Mr. Brown never had kidney problems, yet he now required dialysis. He had just been given a clean bill of health from his doctor earlier in the month, but now on Thursday, July 27, Viewpark Hospital told her that her husband was going to die.

"Mrs. Brown, early in Mr. Brown's hospital stay, wondered how she was going to get him home considering the seven-hour ride to

Atlanta. He was weak, and she worried about getting on the road with him for such a long drive. Now, with this new prognosis, Mrs. Brown was desperate to get him home to Everett, to his own doctors who knew him."

Elizabeth paced in front of the jurors and turned to look directly at them.

"Now, let's return to Tuesday, July 25, day four, when it was discovered that Mr. Brown had RSV and all the antibiotics were stopped. The hematologist made a very important recommendation. He said to hold all anticoagulation medicines—to stop the blood thinners. He also said to monitor for bleeding and, if the patient actively bled, to give him a unit of platelets. Again, he said this on day four, Tuesday, July 25."

Elizabeth repeated the recommendation for emphasis and to give the jurors time to make notes.

"Give the patient one unit of platelets if he bleeds. Monitor him. If you find he's actively bleeding, give him platelets.

"Let's talk about this recommendation made to the hospitalist by his hematology consultant. How do you monitor to determine if the patient is bleeding? One of the tests that should have been done is called FOBT. It means fecal occult blood test, and a piece of stool is put under the microscope to see if there's any microscopic blood in it. It's an easy test, quickly done.

"One of our claims is that Dr. Hamilton should have tested Mr. Brown early for microscopic bleeding because Mr. Brown had four stools on Thursday, July 27, but they did not test at that time when the bleeding could have been detected much earlier. In fact, they never tested at all. I remind you, the hematology consultant said on Tuesday, July

25 to monitor for bleeding. They never monitored for bleeding, as instructed by the hematologist. They never tested for microscopic bleeding at all.

"The reason I want to talk about this is because of what happened on Sunday morning. Remember that Saturday morning, July 29 at 4:30 a.m. was when the nurse found the first black stool. She knew he was bleeding. The nurse called Dr. Chad's service and told his nurse at 6:30 a.m. what she found. Just a couple of hours later, at 8:00 a.m., Mr. Brown produced another black stool. Dr. Chad didn't see Mr. Brown until later at noon, nearly six hours after his office had been notified of the black stools that indicate bleeding, and nearly eight hours after the first bloody stool was found. But before Dr. Chad showed up, the hematologist who wrote the order to monitor the blood and get him platelets came to see Mr. Brown.

"For some reason, the hematologist missed the two black stools and did not document this in the record. However, Dr. Chad *did know* about it. He returned on Saturday from his time off, so as a hospitalist, he was back on duty and responsible for Mr. Brown's care.

"In the meantime, that Sunday morning Mrs. Brown called her daughter-in-law, Marna Marsh, who married her son, Michael. Her father is a doctor, and Mrs. Brown spoke to the doctor to explain what was going on."

Upon Elizabeth saying that, the defense offered an objection, although there should be none during opening arguments.

"That's hearsay, your honor."

"It's not offered to prove the truth of the matter," Elizabeth said.

"Just a moment," the judge said. "Approach the bench."

The attorneys approached the judge, and they huddled there for a few moments. The judge then sent them back.

"There's no testimony," the judge said, "so the objection to hearsay is misplaced. She's only telling the jury what the evidence will be, so I'm not going to consider that testimony. It's not testimony. Overruled."

"Thank you, your honor," Elizabeth said.

I realized I had been holding my breath, and after the ruling, I let it out. I know little about court procedures, and the defense's objection made me wonder what they were up to. I was happy to hear the judge overruled the objection.

Elizabeth continued to explain to the jury that my daughter-in-law's father, a physician, felt from all that I described that Mr. Brown was very sick and that I had nothing to lose by moving him to Everett.

"Dr. Chad decided on Sunday, July 30 to obtain a GI consult, as it was clear from the stools that Thomas was now bleeding in his upper GI tract. But the order was not a 'stat' order, meaning it was not deemed to be urgent. The GI doctor would have seen Mr. Brown within six hours with a stat order. But the GI doctor finally showed up on Sunday, July 30 at noon, thirty-two hours since the first stool was found on Saturday, July 29 at 4:30 a.m.

"Thirty-two hours."

Elizabeth repeated her last statement to make sure it sunk in. "Thirty-two hours passed before the GI doctor finally arrived for the consult while Mr. Brown continued to bleed.

"The GI doctor determined Mr. Brown was not stable enough for the endoscopy that could repair the bleed. Mr. Brown had several issues going on now—acute kidney injury, anemia, confusion, caused by encephalopathy—and he had a feeding tube. And his platelets were low at sixty-one. Hospital policy requires platelets to be at seventy-five for invasive surgery so that a patient will properly clot and not bleed to death during or after surgery.

"Note that one unit of platelets will raise the level of platelets by fifty thousand. So, one unit of platelets would have brought Mr. Brown's platelet count to well above the requirement for surgery.

"In the meantime, the GI doctor prescribed Protonix, which aids in acid damage to the stomach, and wrote a note that the patient could not have the surgery until he was stable. But the GI doctor's notes say more."

Elizabeth put the note up on the screen for everyone to see.

"You can see that the GI doctor noted in the chart that Mr. Brown's platelets were too low, and it was dangerous to do the endoscopy because he wouldn't clot. Once stable, Mr. Brown would require an endoscopy to find the source of the bleeding.

"But Dr. Chad didn't appear to interpret the note to mean that he—the hospitalist, the one in charge, the one who considers all recommendations from consultants and determines the next course of action—should administer the platelets to make Mr. Brown stable for surgery. And it appears he did not clarify who would give the platelets to Mr. Brown—himself or the GI doctor.

"And so, as Mr. Brown continued to bleed, Mr. Brown's platelet count, according to our chart, dropped down to forty-five, forty-two, then forty-one. He never received platelets. He never was scoped.

"Mr. Brown continued to bleed until he died."

Elizabeth paused to let the weight of that horrific fact sink in. It took all I had to keep from crying.

"The GI doctor will say that he verbally spoke to Dr. Chad about the need for platelets as that is his customary practice—to verbally confirm his requirements. But Dr. Chad says the GI doctor never told him this. So, there is a misunderstanding of what's *noted in the chart* about who will give the platelets, as well as the *oral communication* between the hospitalist and the gastroenterologist regarding who will give the platelets.

"And Dr. Chad, the hospitalist who should know what's going on at all times, did not seem to see it as his responsibility to make sure Mr. Brown got the platelets. Dr. Chad will tell you later that he is not the only one who can give platelets, essentially passing the buck. The GI doctor can administer the platelets too. But Dr. Chad, the hospitalist, must ensure there is a meeting of the minds about who is giving the platelets to the patient.

"As time passed, no one, especially Dr. Chad, the hospitalist in charge, seemed to ask the right questions about the status of Mr. Brown, who continued to bleed. Mr. Brown never received the platelets to raise his hemoglobin to a level that would make him a candidate for the endoscopy to stop the bleeding.

"Mr. Brown's bleed was never treated."

Elizabeth walked over to the jury and again gestured to me. She talked about how I communicated with everyone, beginning with the fact that I wanted to move Thomas to Everett. The kidney doctor's notes reflected it. So did the hematologist's notes. The social worker's records reflected it as well, specifically writing that Dr. Chad was going to call Everett to get a doctor to accept Mr. Brown.

"Yet Dr. Chad's records made no mention of Mrs. Brown's wish to transfer Mr. Brown, nor did they mention Dr. Chad's intention to contact Everett. Dr. Chad's notes are devoid of Mrs. Brown's request to move her husband to Everett in Atlanta and devoid of his intention to make the call required of him—the hospitalist—to make that happen."

There it was, laid out at the jury's feet. The truth about what they had done to Thomas. It was almost too much for me to process, to hear it laid out so factually. It is not that I ever had any doubts about what they had done—but the way Elizabeth described it all so succinctly and in language everyone could understand made it seem like it was a new revelation all over again. And it hurt just as much.

But Elizabeth was not finished.

She told the jury how excited we were on Monday, July 31 that we may be able to get Thomas home, how we had set up a GoFundMe specifically because so many family and friends wanted to do something to help us.

"Mrs. Brown will testify how this was a very difficult time for her. How Dr. Chad, after explaining the entire process of the *doctor-to-doctor* transfer of a patient, told *her* that she needed to make the call to make arrangements with Everett. How there was a period of time when she called and did everything she could to make the transfer until someone at Everett finally told her that she could not arrange the transfer. A *doctor* had to make that arrangement by calling and sharing medical information about the patient."

It was then that Elizabeth revealed to the jury that she had obtained recordings of the calls to and from Everett—the first one was after I demanded Dr. Chad call Everett when he refused to make the initial call. I had insisted on listening to Dr. Chad's conversation because I felt I could not trust him to follow through with the call.

Then she dropped another bombshell.

"There's another call later that night that's very important. The call occurs at 7:09 p.m., just after Dr. Chad is off duty. Everett calls Dr. Chad, and there are two conversations. One is when the doctor, after hearing Dr. Chad's description of Mr. Brown, asked if he had been scoped. Dr. Chad said, 'No, the gastroenterologist doesn't think he's stable enough.' They asked why he wasn't stable enough, and Dr. Chad responded that, among other things, Mr. Brown's platelets were too low.

"So, Dr. Chad knew. He knew Mr. Brown needed the platelets. Why didn't he give Mr. Brown the platelets that he needed?

"The Everett doctor then asked in what part of the hospital was Mr. Brown. The Everett doctor wanted to know if Mr. Brown was going to be transferred from Viewpark's ICU to their ICU, or from their lower-level unit to Everett's lower-level unit. When Everett determined that Mr. Brown needed to be in an ICU, the Everett doctor told Dr. Chad that he needed to talk to Viewpark's ICU physician in order to transfer him. Everett's ICU doctor came on the line and also asked Dr. Chad if Mr. Brown was scoped.

"Once again, Dr. Chad said no, due to Mr. Brown's low platelet count. Twice he admitted to knowing about the platelets in his discussions with Everett, though he only focuses on his belief that the gastroenterologist never had a verbal conversation with him about the need to give Mr. Brown platelets."

I was infuriated.

Elizabeth pointed out that at that point in the call, the Everett doctors accepted the transfer, saying that as soon as a bed was available, they would be able to bring Thomas to Everett. She then went on to tell the jury that on the same night, the night nurse at Viewpark called Dr. Zeller, an ICU physician, or intensivist, because Thomas was having trouble. Dr. Zeller said that he would not be admitting Mr. Brown to ICU because he had to be intubated for that to happen, per hospital policy, but they would put him in the ICU area to monitor him more closely. Thomas was placed in ICU unofficially.

As such, Dr. Zeller was never officially his doctor because Thomas was not officially in the ICU. He continued to be under the care of Drs. Chad and Hamilton, and according to them, he was never sick enough for ICU care, despite the serious bleeding.

Elizabeth went on to summarize additional pertinent facts—about how Thomas seemed to stabilize between Sunday and Monday, and how Dr. Chad told me that he should be put in hospice care. That Thomas would only suffer and that he "needed" to be made comfortable.

"Mrs. Brown was put in the position of having to make the most difficult choice of her life," Elizabeth said. "As a couple who loved each other very much, they had talked about what to do if Mr. Brown ever got into a situation where there was no hope—that he didn't want to be kept alive artificially. Mrs. Brown had to decide whether to honor that or keep fighting. And she chose to honor his wishes, and since Dr. Chad said that all of his organs were shutting down and he wasn't going live, she had to let him go."

It was so hard to hear that all again. I fought back tears as Elizabeth talked about what happened at hospice.

"The hospice doctor who admitted Dr. Brown will testify that the admitting diagnosis was acute respiratory failure due to *gastrointestinal bleeding*. She will explain that he had lost sufficient blood over a long period of time—that Mr. Brown had lost a third of his blood volume and that he died early the next morning. She will explain that her diagnosis for cause of death was acute gastric *hemorrhaging*. She signed a death certificate, and it was the same as her admitting diagnosis.

"Mrs. Brown decided to do an autopsy to find out exactly what happened. Dr. Wallace Armstrong performed an independent exam and found a large bleeding ulcer penetrating through an artery, and it filled his small intestines and large intestines with blood. His colon was three times the size it should have been, also full of blood. Plus, the administration of some medications issued to him made his respirations go down. He had no reserves to fight his condition.

"Dr. Armstrong also found a mucus plug in Mr. Brown's lower left lung, and the expert witnesses believe that this plug was causing the breathing situation—a condition that's not fatal or terminal. They treat it by sticking a tube down your nose and suctioning it out. If they had ordered the CAT scan that morning, as advised by the pulmonologist, they would have seen it and resolved the issue.

"So, we have brought this action on behalf of Mrs. Brown. We allege that Dr. Hamilton was negligent for not testing for blood earlier that week. Had he tested Mr. Brown's stools earlier and monitored Mr. Brown, the microscopic bleeding would have been discovered by Friday, or sooner, many hours earlier than the discovery of the black stool. The gastroenterologist could have done the scope, found the bleed, and stopped it. Everyone agrees that if they stopped the bleed, Mr. Brown would not have died."

Though she tried to stay calm, I could hear the frustration in Elizabeth's voice rising. Her tone became sharper. She stared intensely at the members of the jury.

"Each of our experts will testify that Mr. Brown could have been saved on Friday, Saturday, Sunday, Monday, or Tuesday had they stopped the bleed by a procedure that takes anywhere from seven to thirty minutes, depending on what they find. The GI doctor came to see him all three days. He came on Sunday and said he wasn't stable enough for the procedure. He came on Monday and said he still wasn't stable enough but that he was being transferred to Everett. They gave him a transfusion then because they said Mr. Brown would need blood before he left for Everett. He came again on Tuesday but got notice that Mr. Brown was in hospice. Once hospice was involved, there was no more aggressive treatment.

"That meant no more dialysis. No more transfusions. He was without everything that had been supporting him. It all stopped. We're alleging that Dr. Chad should have given him platelets once they knew what the problem was. Just one unit of platelets would have been enough for the GI doctor to fix the bleed. Dr. Chad's failure to give that one unit of platelets was negligent. We allege that he knew that's all that was needed, and he didn't do it. It was his job, because he's the only one on this team who knew everything all of the other doctors said, and he coordinated all care. He knew what needed to be done.

"Additionally, our expert Dr. Sherry will testify that Mr. Brown did not need to be sent to hospice—that he should have been sent to the ICU for treatment. Mr. Brown was initially admitted to the standard floor, moved to PCU, the step-up unit, but never moved to ICU. ICU was wrongfully bypassed when Mr. Brown was sent to hospice. He says that Mr. Brown's organs were *not* shutting down, that they were no different than the day before, that this was a negligent referral to hospice, and that the patient should have been actively treated in ICU.

"Ladies and gentlemen, this is something Mrs. Brown had to learn after we investigated this case, and let me tell you, that's a hard thing to learn—that the person you love most in life didn't have to die. This chapter is the last chapter of this story, and it will be written here this week in this courtroom."

Elizabeth thanked the members of the jury for their service, as well as everyone else in the room. The judge then ordered a brief recess to straighten up the courtroom and allow the setup of materials for the opening statement by the defense.

All told, Elizabeth's remarks took approximately ninety minutes. Her presence was mesmerizing. She had my complete focus the entire time, and not just because of the way she spoke. That was the first time I had heard the complete story summarized in that way. I had heard all the pieces over time, but to hear them put together, to understand how all those pieces fit—it was devastating to know that Thomas's life could have been saved at, quite literally, any point in time during his hospital stay.

As I listened to Elizabeth, I watched the jury, assessing whether or not they comprehended all she was telling them. Some seemed quite sharp and took notes throughout her statement. Others just watched her. I worried about them because there was so much information to take in that I wondered if it was too much for them. Would they understand the major points she made about the administration of platelets and how necessary they were to the lifesaving surgery Thomas needed?

When she returned to our table, Elizabeth took my hand and squeezed it. I squeezed back and saw she was just as drained as I was. She threw 150 percent of herself into these cases and left no stone unturned in her opening argument. She went into so much detail so that the jury could see what Thomas had gone through day by day, moment by moment, as he struggled to live.

I just hoped it would be enough.

CHAPTER 17

THE DEFENSE OPENS

ONCE WE HAD EATEN AND REFRESHED, WE RETURNED TO THE
courtroom for the defense's opening statements.

Similar to Elizabeth, the defense had a PowerPoint presentation
and medical notes that they put up on a screen. Mr. Cooper, the lead
defense attorney, stood up from his table and faced the jury.

"Good afternoon. My name is Conner Cooper, and with my partners,
it's our honor in this case to represent Viewpark Hospital, Dr. Colin
Chad, and Dr. Samuel Hamilton.

"On July 6, 2017, Mr. Brown went into a walk-in clinic in Atlanta and
told them he thought he was sick, and that he thought there was a problem with his kidneys. Twenty-two days later, his kidneys had failed. He
couldn't eat. He couldn't swallow. He couldn't eat ice chips. He had a
temperature that spiked to 105.

"And all of this was before there was ever a GI bleed. In fact, it was the
condition that caused those symptoms that caused the GI bleed. Mr.

Brown developed a virus sometimes called an RSV virus, and it caused several problems for him.

"Let's look at these things in terms of cause and effect. Cause and effect is a 105 degree temperature and Mr. Brown's kidneys not working. He couldn't make urine. They had to put him on dialysis so he could make urine. He gained—literally—fifty pounds of weight while he was in the hospital at Viewpark because they were putting so much water into his body, to try to keep his equilibrium because of what this virus had done to his system. And they couldn't get that weight off—even with the dialysis.

"We're going to go through all the doctors that were involved in this case, as well as all the nurses and respiratory therapists. But after twenty months of litigating this case, you'll see there are two very important healthcare providers—speech pathologists who came in on July 28, before there was a GI bleed, and did an evaluation. They did this because Dr. Chad asked them to, because he saw that Mr. Brown was having a hard time. He couldn't even swallow his own secretions.

"So, the speech pathologists came in. They're specialists, and you'll hear from them the tests they performed to determine if he could even swallow—and it wasn't a physical issue. It was because he had encephalopathy. His brain wasn't working to allow him to swallow properly. Again, he couldn't even swallow ice chips. They put them in his mouth, and they couldn't even manipulate his tongue correctly to do that.

"The next day, he got even worse. Another speech pathologist came in, and he couldn't swallow *anything*. At that point in time, they had to put a feeding tube in him because he couldn't feed himself. He also had a drop in hemoglobin. We're going to look at a chart about that. The fact is that his hemoglobin went down all because of the effects of the virus—all before a GI bleed had happened.

"What else did this virus cause? Well, it actually caused the GI bleed. His medications *may* have had some minor contribution, but they were minimal. He took aspirin three times, Advil three times, and one dose of IV contrast for a CT scan they *had* to perform. All of this was due to the virus.

"As a result, Mr. Brown developed what is called a stress ulcer. These things are common in the hospital. So, what you're going to see—what the evidence is going to show as we go through it—is that ultimately, by the time the GI bleed started on the twenty-eighth, the damage was already done to his system at that time and, unfortunately, he was never going to be able to recover from it.

"Mr. Brown had a respiratory virus. A virus is not bacteria. You heard a lot about antibiotics. Antibiotics are totally ineffective against the virus. The only thing that ever showed up on any testing was this virus, not bacteria. You've heard about covering things empirically, and that's what the doctors did because they weren't sure until they got the results. Then, one infectious disease doctor came in and ordered a test, a nasal swab for the RSV, and it came back positive. Until that time, all other cultures were negative. Before then, they thought maybe—in fact, you'll see it throughout the records—that maybe Mr. Brown had a urinary tract infection from when he was in Georgia.

"But what we found out after we got the records from the Georgia walk-in clinic was that they performed a urinalysis, and it turned out to be negative. And they tried to call the Browns and just never got through. So, they never knew that. When they got to Orlando, they told the hospital that they thought Mr. Brown had a UTI. That's why it's in all the records all the time. That's why it's in Dr. Chad's records, because the doctor took a history from the patient who thought he had a UTI. Again, the urinalysis at the Georgia walk-in clinic was negative, but the Browns apparently never knew that. Also, the urinalysis performed at

Viewpark Hospital came up negative. The only thing that ever came up positive was this RSV virus.

"And this is the key. There can be consequences of a viral infection that last even after you eliminate the fever. That's what you're going to hear in this case from the plaintiff. They're going to say the fever was all gone. Their argument is that they stopped the antibiotics, so there must have been no infection.

"But you don't treat a virus with antibiotics, so that wouldn't matter. *That's* why they stopped the antibiotics—because they figured out it was a virus, not bacteria. When a virus attacks the body's immune systems, it starts the process that raises the temperature, and you'll see his white blood cell counts, when he first came in, went low and later went way high. That can lead to organ failure—kidneys, brain, and breathing.

"You're going to hear from experts that the RSV virus in the last ten years has become a very serious problem in the elderly, particularly in places like nursing homes. Now, it's true that children under age two can also get the virus and they can be treated for it pretty easily and it goes away. But for some reason, this virus has gotten to the point where for the elderly it is very difficult to manage, giving them what they call in legal terms a high morbidity and mortality. That means it can cause problems and can cause death."

It took everything I had to keep from fidgeting in my seat. It was difficult to sit still with little expression on my face, as instructed by Elizabeth, while the defense attorney drew unsound conclusions and twisted the truth. In just the first few minutes of his opening statement, he had said that Thomas had RSV that caused the bleed and that is why he died.

I thought, *Let's suppose RSV caused the bleed. Still, fix the bleed! Is he saying Thomas had RSV, therefore they must let him bleed to death?*

This was so illogical to me, and I hoped that the jurors would see it the same way.

He continued, "So, my opening statement is going to be a little bit of a road map for you all, to try to help you put together the evidence that you're going to hear. I'm going to try to tell you what we expect the evidence to show. There are some principles that you should be guided by in looking at this case and how you make your decision.

"Listen to the whole story. You heard my colleague tell you in *voir dire* that the plaintiff has to go first. There are psychological studies that basically say that people tend to believe more what they listen to first, but in our jury process, the way that the rules have been developed, you're not supposed to make up your mind until you hear all of the evidence and go back to the jury room. We go second. So, we're a little behind from the beginning. But the rules tell you that you should listen to the whole story before making up your mind.

"Number two, common sense. You've probably heard the phrase before to not check your common sense at the door. Always bring your common sense to bear in making decisions.

"Number three, sympathy. You've heard about that. You have a jury instruction on that. No one is asking anyone not to have sympathy, but you must set it aside in making your decision and decide on the facts and the evidence. The burden of proof in this case is on the plaintiff.

"Their allegation in this case is that based on Mr. Armstrong's autopsy, Mr. Brown died of a GI bleed and that Dr. Chad and Dr. Hamilton were negligent. And we'll talk about Dr. Chad for a minute. He's board-certified as a family medicine hospitalist. You've heard already that hospitalists typically come from one of two branches of medicine. There are internal medicine doctors and there are family medicine doctors. Generally, a hospitalist is one of the two.

"Dr. Chad is not board-certified in internal medicine because he's not an internal medicine doctor. He's a family medicine doctor, and he's board-certified for that. He grew up and went to medical school abroad and then came to the United States mainland to do his medical training, his residency, which is after medical school. He did that at Ohio State University. And then, importantly, he also did what's called a fellowship, which is additional training, in geriatrics, which is taking care of people in the geriatric population. He's published numerous articles for the Journal of the American Geriatric Society.

"Dr. Hamilton *is* an internal medicine doctor. He's what's called an osteopathic doctor, which is a different kind of medicine—a DO instead of an MD. He did his internal medicine residency at the University of North Texas."

The mention of those names made my jaw tighten. To hear Mr. Cooper speak about them as though they were these consummate professionals to be revered by the jury was offensive. *It doesn't matter what their credentials are if they don't care enough about the patient to provide the best of care.*

Mr. Cooper went on to explain to the jury that though they would hear about the many nurses and specialists who were called in to consult on Thomas's care, none of them were accused of negligence and were not considered defendants in the case. He explained the differences in nephrology, hematology, gastroenterology, and pulmonology, as well as what an intensivist was. He then put a list on the screen detailing the key medical personnel involved in the case, as well as which ones had been deposed by Elizabeth and whose recorded depositions the jury would watch via video.

"What the plaintiffs have to do," Mr. Cooper continued, "is to prove negligence—a deviation from the appropriate standard of care by Dr. Chad and Dr. Hamilton. You'll also get a jury instruction about what that means. They have to prove causation, and you'll get an instruction about what that means as well. Also, the issue in this case is one of non-economic damages. Mrs. Faiella has said Mrs. Brown suffers from lack of companionship from Mr. Brown. There is no claim in this case for what are called economic damages. There's no claim for medical bills.

"You heard Mr. Brown was retired. Mrs. Brown, I believe, is now retired. There's no claim for lost wages or lost support services. This is a non-economic damages case. We're not lessening that—we just want to make sure you're clear that this is not a case of economic damages. So, I have this calendar here, and actually, I think as time goes along, you'll probably see Mrs. Faiella has a nice one too. I think they had to do theirs on the fly because they forgot it."

Mr. Cooper was making reference to the fact that despite all of Elizabeth's preparation with slides and other examples, she had used a hand-drawn calendar to mark the timeline of events. His jab dripped with sarcasm and was clearly designed to get the jury to dislike Elizabeth or to make her seem less competent in some way. The effort was a reach at best, and I hoped that my growing distaste for this man was not apparent on my face.

"At any rate, the calendar here is important because, as I said, we believe the evidence is going to show that Mr. Brown had suffered significant consequences to his body, none of them being caused by the bleed that ultimately led to his death."

Mr. Cooper then went into Thomas's health history. He talked about the fact that Thomas had a cough for two weeks. That he had a history of hypertension and diabetes, though he left out, of course, that Thomas had well managed them both. He pointed out that Thomas had been treated with radiation for his prostate cancer. He talked about his peripheral vascular stents and his history of smoking, and while he admitted that Thomas quit the habit over twenty years prior, he also pointed out that physicians will say that extensive smoking will have long-term effects, even after quitting.

Essentially, he ignored the fact that Thomas was in good health before he came to the hospital. He was doing everything he could to paint a picture for the jury that Thomas was a frail seventy-four-year-old man who was susceptible to this virus and that it was that illness, not the negligence of Dr. Chad and Dr. Hamilton, that ultimately led to his death. The implication made me tightly clasp my hands and put all of my energy there so that my face showed no expression.

With that picture in the jury's mind, Mr. Cooper then went down the chain of events much in the way Elizabeth had. I hated to admit how effective his tactic had been. Listing all of the issues Thomas had to deal with physically prior to this situation made it seem perfectly reasonable to people who did not know that Thomas was, in fact, healthy that he could succumb to something like RSV.

While I had every confidence in Elizabeth, as Mr. Cooper went through the horrible events all over again, I became anxious. There was no getting around it—the defense was crafty. Mr. Cooper knew that this jury was made up of individuals with no medical background. I had to admit that, had I been sitting in that jury box, I would not have known who to believe.

Mr. Cooper continued his argument by talking about Thomas's hemoglobin and how their experts would testify that the virus, not the GI bleed, was responsible for the change in levels. He also explained the differences in sepsis—blood infections—caused by bacteria versus sepsis caused by a virus. He then shifted the focus to Dr. Hamilton.

"Let me talk for a moment about Dr. Hamilton. You've heard the allegation of negligence against Dr. Hamilton, about the fact that he did not order what's called a fecal occult blood test in the hospital. There was no reason for him to do that at that point in time, according to our experts, and you'll hear them talk about that. In fact, all of the stools—and this is something not very nice to talk about—but in the hospital, nurses monitor all of your different systems, including your stool.

"So, the nurses monitor stools, and you'll see their records of all of the days in this time frame. There was one day when Mr. Brown had three stools, all normal. Then a day and a half before the bleed, at about midnight, he had a normal stool. Dr. Hamilton allegedly didn't order a fecal occult blood test in that time frame—when all the stools were normal."

As I said—he was crafty. Mr. Cooper knew how to twist things just enough to make you doubt what you thought you knew. He emphasized "normal stools," hoping the jurors would not recall that stools may appear normal to the naked eye although there was microscopic blood in them. Plus, the blood tests were indicating that Thomas was losing blood, so the stools should have been tested.

Mr. Cooper continued to make the case that all of the symptoms Thomas experienced were due to complications from the RSV and not negligence on the parts of Dr. Chad and Dr. Hamilton. Then we reached the point in the timeline where Thomas should have been transferred to the intensive care unit.

"So, there's an issue in this case about moving the patient to the ICU. At this point in time, Mr. Brown was on what they call a regular floor, or a PCU floor. The nurses had the intensivist, Dr. Zeller, come to see Mr. Brown due to his declining condition. Dr. Zeller is the one who would have been able to say, 'Let's get this man to the ICU.' They did not do that. Why?

"Because the evidence will show that patients who need to go to the ICU have to meet certain criteria—one of the main ones being that they have to be intubated. And we've all seen that Mr. Brown was not. So, what did they do? They moved him to the ICU unit, but they couldn't put him in what's called *intensive care* because he wasn't intubated."

I asked Elizabeth about this criterion before the trial. "Is this a medical protocol?" She told me no, that it was only a protocol for the *hospital*. This limited and inadequate criteria for moving a patient to ICU did not consider other situations warranting ICU care, like excessive bleeding.

To me, that is a problem with the policy. In other hospitals, a patient does not have to be intubated to be referred to the ICU. Of course, Mr. Cooper did not differentiate between medical protocol and hospital protocol, so it was possible that the jurors were unaware of the issues that this ICU criteria created.

At that point, Mr. Cooper turned his argument to the issue of the stress ulcer.

"This is going to be the point where we're going to get to laugh at my artistic skill, because I'm a pretty bad artist," he said, getting a few smiles out of the jurors. "I'm going to try to draw a little bit where this bleed was."

Mr. Cooper began sketching on a poster board. "You have an esophagus, which is where the food comes down from the mouth, then the stomach, and then you have the small intestines, which run for quite a ways. And this bleed is right in here." He waved a hand over his crude drawing. "When the autopsy was done, they found a number of different areas throughout here that had a little erosion. The one you've heard about is penetrating, which is a little misleading because there wasn't a hole that went all the way through. If there *was* a hole that went all the way through, the contents would have spilled into his cavity, and he would have gotten even sicker than he was. That didn't happen.

"So that leads to an important point in this case. Dr. Chad called in the gastroenterologist about the melanotic stool. Again, this is not the nicest thing to talk about, but it is important. The stool is described as black and tarry. Why is that? Because when you have a bleed and it starts coming all the way through there, that's the color it turns when there's a slow bleed. That's what you see."

I wanted to jump right up out of my seat. Mr. Cooper had contradicted himself with his own argument! He had just finished telling the jury that the process starts way up in the intestines, so by the time it comes out in the stool, the person has been bleeding for a *while*.

Sadly, I knew that this was all so much for the jury to understand, let alone to pick up on something like that without having it pointed out to them in the moment—and Mr. Cooper knew it too. In fact, I am sure he was counting on it.

"This is important. Look at each part of this. This is a seventy-four-year-old man with multiple medical problems, including sepsis, bronchitis, acute kidney injury and chronic kidney disease, anemia, pancytopenia, metabolic acidosis, encephalopathy, and dysphagia."

Once again, he was making Thomas out to be this sick, unhealthy individual, completely ignoring the fact that Thomas did not have *any* of those conditions when he entered the hospital. *The doctors at that hospital created those conditions!* Thomas had a slight temperature, and they initially treated it by pumping him full of antibiotics and medications that caused bleeding ulcers. They shut his kidneys down without properly monitoring him. They gave him several blood thinners when he already had blood thinners in his system. *Those* actions created all the conditions Mr. Cooper had just listed. But he wasn't going to tell that part of the story—that was on us.

"The allegation in this case is that Dr. Chad did not give Mr. Brown platelets to raise his levels high enough to allow the gastroenterologist to perform an endoscopy to determine the source of the bleed. When you hear the GI doctor's testimony, you'll hear that he felt that all of his reasons for not performing the endoscopy were his own, not Dr. Chad's. He's not getting sued in this case, yet he feels these decisions were his own. He decided not to do the endoscopy because he felt the patient wasn't stable enough—that the patient might not even make it through the procedure."

What Mr. Cooper failed to mention—or rather, chose not to—was the fact that the GI doctor's notes were unclear, something Elizabeth would later call greater attention to. The GI doctor only indicated the current state of Thomas's condition, and that when Thomas became stable, he could perform the endoscopy. He never specifically explained to Dr. Chad that platelets must be given to make Thomas stable. And Dr. Chad, who did not effectively analyze the information the GI doctor gave him, never concluded on his own that stabilizing Thomas meant administering platelets.

"Let's step back a little bit and look at the issue of the patient dying. Their contention is that the patient died of a GI bleed. Every expert in this case has been asked, 'Was this patient in hemodynamic shock at the time he died?' No, he wasn't. In fact, his blood pressure and vital signs were generally within a somewhat normal range during that time frame. His organs were shutting down.

"So, when making the decision to go to hospice, there's a process you have to go through with this. They sent a nurse over to evaluate the record, to talk to the hospice doctor, and then determine if a patient is an appropriate candidate for hospice. And they did. They accepted Mr. Brown into hospice."

I struggled to remain expressionless. Dr. Chad had convinced me that hospice was the only option, not ICU—but I remembered Elizabeth's advice to let her be the lawyer, to let her try the case. It was going to be hard, once on the stand, to not point out all these discrepancies. It was going to be a struggle for me to not argue the case myself.

"This is a note you're going to see from the hospital chaplain after Dr. Chad had talked to Mrs. Brown. This, of course, is not an easy discussion for any person or patient's relative to have. Of course not. It's a difficult decision. The chaplain's notation of his conversation was Mrs. Brown said, 'I don't want this. I'm ready for hospice.'"

What!? That simply was not true.

I may have said, "I don't want this." I can see myself saying that. I was traumatized. I was told my husband was sick. He was dying. If I said that, what I meant was, "I don't want this situation to be. I don't want my husband to die." Never did I say *anything* about hospice. Hospice did not come up until Dr. Chad brought it up to me days later. Why would I offer up hospice?

My stepdaughter, Nichelle, had called the chaplain. She needed to speak to him. I never said the word "hospice" while the chaplain was there or at all. The only thing I could think of is that the records might have been altered, like Elizabeth had suggested during our very first contact.

Mr. Cooper continued.

"The GI doctor came to see the patient on August 1 and didn't seem to be too upset that this patient might be bleeding out and that they were sending a bleeding out patient to hospice."

At that, Elizabeth stood.

"Objection, your honor. Approach the bench?" The judge motioned for both sides to approach. Elizabeth explained, "This is the argument that the GI doctor didn't do anything—that his hair wasn't on fire. This is the argument we've already discussed, which is to say that there was inaction on the part of the GI doctor, implying that it's okay for there to be inaction on the part of Dr. Chad. This is exactly the motion in limine that the court ruled on. It's an argument in an opening statement."

"I'm not arguing that the GI doctor did anything wrong," Mr. Cooper said. "I'm saying *no one* did anything wrong. This is all relevant evidence as to why these other gentlemen, the other specialists regarding the GI bleed and blood platelets, did not find there to be any problem with sending the patient to hospice. That is relevant evidence in this case to rebut the plaintiff's allegation that Dr. Chad was negligent by sending the patient to hospice."

"Exact same argument," Elizabeth said.

"Objection sustained."

"Thank you, your honor," Elizabeth said.

Both attorneys returned to their respective tables. Mr. Cooper did not appear to like being checked. He moved quickly through the list of witnesses to be called who would either discredit our case or prove how their testimony would support theirs. Then he went into details about the calls between Everett and Dr. Chad, and how it was clear from the recording of the call that Dr. Chad wanted to help Thomas get into their ICU, but Everett simply did not have the bed at the time. That notion infuriated me, and I could not wait to hear that recording.

Mr. Cooper continued on, talking about his expert witness: a physician who disagreed with Dr. Armstrong's assessment of the mucus plug found in Thomas's lung and what that meant for his condition. It seems Dr. Armstrong had not sent out the mucus plug for fungal testing, which would have indicated organ shutdown, but by the time the defense's expert had raised this issue, it was too late for Dr. Armstrong to perform the test retroactively. Mr. Cooper reminded the jurors of the differences of opinion regarding the RSV and its contribution to Thomas's death. He then stated that Dr. Armstrong had never reviewed the hospital records prior to performing the autopsy and that, in his deposition, he admitted that he did not know Thomas had tested positive for RSV.

Mr. Cooper was trying to discredit Dr. Armstrong's autopsy findings.

The looks on the jurors' faces were ones of surprise. It was clear that this piece of information—Dr. Armstong being unaware of Thomas's RSV diagnosis—hit home with them. It did not go unnoticed by Mr. Cooper either.

"You get to judge their credibility," Mr. Cooper said. "So, folks, I'm certainly taking longer than I intended. Thank you so much for your attention. Thank you for your service as jurors. We hope when you hear all the evidence and look at it, you will see that you should not be swayed by sympathy. When you look at the totality of the evidence, you will see that Mr. Brown had a GI bleed, but he did not die because of the GI bleed. Thank you very much."

As Mr. Cooper returned to his desk, I seethed, angry as much for what he did not say as for what he did. He faulted Dr. Armstrong for not reviewing the hospital records or performing those tests, but he said nothing of the fact that Dr. Chad and Dr. Zeller refused to obtain Thomas's medical records from Everett to determine how to best treat him. He claimed that Thomas did not die from a GI bleed but left out the fact that the hospice doctor who signed Thomas's death certificate indicated that he died of hemorrhagic gastritis. The hospice doctor was to be respected for deeming Thomas to be appropriate for hospice, yet her diagnosis of the cause of death was not to be believed.

I had this nagging feeling that the defense was putting forth a simple case that was easy for a person to understand, especially a person who might not have been able to grasp all of the intricate medical details of the case. The defense even arbitrarily changed the cause of death to RSV to accommodate their easy explanation. I had seen enough of Mr. Cooper's maneuvering to know that he was capable of doing anything to win this case—and I did not have a good feeling about what was to come.

Though Elizabeth dismissed what they said and indicated she was not worried in the slightest, I remained concerned. The defense omitted many of the relevant facts, and the manner in which they did so had a good chance of sticking in the minds of the jury because they had made the information so easy to comprehend.

Getting justice for Thomas was going to be a fight.

CHAPTER 18

BELOW THE STANDARD OF CARE

On Friday, November 15, we arrived in the courtroom and again received a warning from the judge that she was concerned about the amount of time that was spent on jury selection and opening statements. We were all feeling the pressure from her consistent announcements about the inability to extend this trial.

Then the judge made another announcement that was shocking—one we had not anticipated.

One of the jurors—Number Three, who had previously filed a lawsuit and who we felt would vote in our favor—had to drop out because of a medical emergency with her husband. That meant that the young woman who was previously designated as the alternate was now a permanent member of the jury. Not only that, but we also only had a week to finish this case, so there was no room for any other issues with jurors. The situation added additional pressure to the consistent warnings about finishing this case on time.

With that warning and a changing jury at the forefront of our minds, Elizabeth called Dr. Hiram Sherry, one of our expert witnesses, to the stand.

Dr. Sherry said that he was a physician specializing in internal medicine, with more than two decades of experience supporting all systems of the body. As a hospitalist, he explained, he worked continuously in the clinic, not in an office.

Dr. Sherry currently worked at NorthShore University and NorthShore Hospital and Academic Medical Center in Detroit, where residents, interns, and many others were constantly going through training. He was a board-certified physician, meaning that he had the most current medical knowledge, so he was often responsible for training residents.

In addition, Dr. Sherry explained how a hospitalist like him works with more than five hundred doctors at the one thousand–bed hospital. He might call on other specialists for their opinions on a case, but he was the center of the process and made all decisions. Consultants would give their opinions to him, but he would be the one to make a decision, put in the orders, and treat the patient.

"Is there a difference between internal medicine and the specialty of family medicine?" Elizabeth asked. I knew she was getting at the fact that Dr. Chad was a family medicine physician, not an internal medicine specialist.

"There is a difference. Family medicine treats a different group than we do. They treat adults like we do, but they also treat children. They treat women for GYN-related issues. We just do adult medicine."

"Do you, as a hospitalist, retain control of your patients after you send them to the ICU?"

"Absolutely. Yes."

"And do you continue to take care of them in the ICU?"

"It depends. Sometimes we are the consultants for the ICU, like a surgery ICU where the surgeon may be the main doctor and we'll be the consultants. But yes, we do take care of patients in the ICU."

"Is there, to your knowledge, a limitation on the ICU only being available to persons who are intubated with a tube in their throat?"

"So, you're referring to what we call ventilation—putting someone on a breathing machine. The answer to that question is no. A patient can go to the ICU without being on a breathing machine. There are some patients who, if their lungs fail, need to be put on a breathing machine, and they go to the ICU, but there are other people who are just sick and need more care."

"Doctor, you've been retained in this case. You reviewed the care given by Viewpark Hospital and by two hospitalists, Dr. Hamilton and Dr. Chad, is that correct?" Dr. Sherry agreed. "Do you have opinions about that care?" Again, he said yes. "And do you have opinions about the cause of Mr. Brown's death?" He confirmed that he did. "Have you done this kind of review in other cases?"

Dr. Sherry said that he had; for approximately ten years or more, he had given testimony in courts of law about his opinions concerning care and causes of death. He had given depositions and gone to trial on at least fifteen separate occasions.

"And have your opinions ever been rejected or disqualified?"

"No. Never."

"Have you provided opinions for the healthcare providers in defense of a case?"

"I have. Sometimes I provide my opinions as support for the doctors or the hospitals who provided care, if they've done what I think they should have. I'll provide my opinion about care for the plaintiff's family, the patient's family. It depends on the case. I support the facts, and so I would support whichever side where I feel the facts are."

"Do you have an approximate ratio of how many times you have testified or given opinions in the favor of the patient and how many times in favor of the doctor?"

"Over my career, about half and half."

"Why do you do this work?"

"I started doing this work because I was looking at care at our own hospital—"

Mr. Cooper stood. "Objection, your honor. Self-serving."

Before Elizabeth could even counter the objection, the judge overruled it. This objection was the first of many that seemed to be nothing more than an attempt by the defense to interrupt the witness and run out the clock, knowing we had a limited number of days in which to complete the trial.

Dr. Sherry continued, "I started doing this work because I was looking at care in our own hospital when things went in a direction that wasn't good and had a bad result. The whole goal of this is to improve our care, so we give feedback to doctors if they make mistakes."

"Objection," Mr. Cooper said again. "This has nothing to do with the testimony in this case."

"Overruled."

Mr. Cooper sat back down again but was still determined to distract from the expert's testimony. Dr. Sherry continued his explanation about how his work has impacted care in their own hospital and how he realized he can have an impact that goes beyond caring for the patients—that he could change systems and change care.

"Objection, your honor. Narrative answer not related at all to the circumstances in this case."

"Overruled."

Elizabeth contained a smile in response to the judge's rapid overruling. She then continued, "Do you have any special area of interest that you have pursued in your profession?"

"Yes. I have an interest in another area, and this is to prevent and treat blood clots. I go around the country teaching other doctors about how to identify blood clots in patients, how to prevent strokes in patients, and how to treat patients with blood thinners. I've given hundreds of lectures across the country and have done research in the area. I've done projects in my own hospital to improve our blood clot and stroke rate, and I've taken some national positions."

Elizabeth asked all the right questions. It seemed to me that even someone without an understanding of all the complex terminology from the opening statements would still see quite clearly that Dr. Sherry was eminently qualified, at the top of his field and recognized by hospitals and professional organizations nationwide. Some of my nervousness subsided—at least for the moment.

"Doctor, have you come to opinions concerning the basic issues in this case?"

"I have."

"Are you able, doctor, to break down very simply the main issues that you focused on when reviewing this case?"

"Yes. There was a reasonable period of time that Mr. Brown was in the hospital and was bleeding. There's no doubt in my mind he was bleeding. We know the blood count had fallen and he bled through his stomach, and that happened throughout the hospital stay. The second issue in this case is that, in my opinion, there's no denying that they could have fixed it. They could have found where the bleeding was. They could have performed a camera procedure like an endoscopy and fixed it."

Mr. Cooper stood again. "Objection, your honor. May we approach?" The judge waved both sides forward. The attorneys hovered around the bench for some time, but I was unable to hear what they said. Whatever it was, it did not work out in the defense's favor. When the judge spoke again, I did my best to keep from smiling.

"Objection is overruled."

"Thank you, your honor," Elizabeth said. "Now, doctor, we were going through the three issues you identified in this case. I think you said that there was bleeding in his stomach."

"Yes, he was bleeding, and that led to his death."

"And you feel that the bleed could have been addressed?"

"Yes, they could have fixed the bleeding. Absolutely."

"And the third thing answered was that nothing prevented them from fixing it. There was nothing that prevented them from using a camera and looking down there. Is that correct?"

"There's one more thing," he said. "The theory that Mr. Brown would have died anyway—I disagree with that."

"So, what do you believe was the cause of death?"

"He died because of a stomach bleed, a GI bleed. And that led to problems with his breathing, because he didn't have enough blood to take the oxygen throughout his body. His blood count was falling, and that indicated that blood was going somewhere. We also know he had blood in his stools on Saturday, July 29, when Dr. Chad returned, and that he had a substantial amount of blood in his stools the next morning. If they had looked earlier than the twenty-ninth and done a blood fecal test, they would have seen there was blood there. They also could have done a fecal occult test earlier, when his counts were falling, to look for microscopic blood in his stool—when you can't see it with the naked eye, but you might suspect there's bleeding."

Dr. Sherry was sharp. He was not content to give short answers. He wanted the jury to understand what he was saying and why it was important. With each answer, I felt more and more confident about his testimony and the effect it might have. If the jury was truly listening, there was no way they could miss these facts.

Elizabeth questioned Dr. Sherry further about whether or not he was familiar with an endoscopy and the particulars of the procedure. Once again, he explained it in simple terms, how the camera is used to find the bleed in a process that takes approximately twenty minutes or less; how they can use a laser on the tip of the camera to zap—or cauterize— the injured blood vessel, effectively halting a life-threatening condition. Some jurors nodded their heads. They understood.

"So, once again, doctor, do you have an opinion as to whether or not, if they had performed the endoscopy and found the bleed, if it could have been fixed?"

"Yes. It could have been fixed. Had they gone down with a camera, it could have been fixed. They needed a few things to make this happen. One of those things is the platelet count. When you call a GI doctor to do that kind of procedure, they have requirements. The platelet level must be at a certain number. They tell the hospitalists to give the patient platelets by hooking them up to an IV and infusing them with platelets until the GI doctor is satisfied enough with the count that he can perform the procedure. The hospitalist should tell the GI doctor that the patient is ready, and the platelets are there. That's what needed to happen in this case—and it didn't happen."

Elizabeth took a moment for the words to sink in with the jury, then pressed on. "Do you have an opinion as to what happened to the patient with regards to why he was first admitted and why he was treated?"

"Yes. He had some weakness and what he thought was a cold. He went to the hospital, and they admitted him. They thought he picked up some kind of virus or flu. They gave him antibiotics in case he had an infection in his lungs. Essentially, he got antibiotics and he was doing okay, and then a few days later his blood counts started to fall."

"And at that point, when the counts started to fall, what should have happened?"

"They should have been asking why his blood count was falling. And that's where the problem occurred, at approximately day four, after he got admitted. The blood count started to fall."

"There was a time when they figured out what was causing that cold?"

"Yes. On day five, they found a virus in his system called RSV. Essentially, it's like a cold, and you don't do anything for this. You prescribe rest, and it goes away. Initially, they were giving him antibiotics thinking he had pneumonia, like a bacterium that needed treatment, but they found out on day five that it was just a virus. He didn't need any of those antibiotics for a virus. He just needed rest."

Elizabeth again paused to let Dr. Sherry's words sink in. I was thrilled at how plainly he explained everything. The facts, to me, seemed incontrovertible. Surely, the jury realized this too. They just had to.

"Okay. Mr. Brown had some normal stools, right? Why wouldn't the bleeding be seen when he had four stools on Thursday? Why would they look normal?"

"The reason you cannot see the bleed is because initially bleeding is microscopic. It's not full bleeding—it's slow bleeding. But at this point, with the blood counts falling, they should be testing for bleeding. That's when they would have used the fecal occult test. That's what should have happened on Thursday, July 27."

Elizabeth did this throughout the trial—asking the next question so that the witness further expounded on the issue, presenting all of the relevant facts in a simple manner. I did not realize it, but I was holding my breath as Dr. Sherry explained so clearly what had happened.

"I would like to ask you whether or not you have an opinion as to whether Dr. Hamilton, Dr. Chad's partner, fell below the standard of care at any time during the twenty-fifth through the twenty-eighth, when he was covering for Dr. Chad?"

"Yes. Remember, the blood count was starting to fall and continued to do so. By Friday, the twenty-eighth, his count was really low. When it started to fall, when Dr. Hamilton took over on Tuesday, July 25, this is where he should have checked for microscopic blood shortly thereafter, as dictated by the hematologist who saw Mr. Brown that day. Dr. Hamilton could have done that over any one of the next couple of days. But he didn't do that."

"So, what happened on Saturday, the twenty-ninth?"

"The twenty-ninth is where Mr. Brown had four or five stools in the morning, dark ones. Dr. Hamilton finally ordered the fecal blood test that morning and they found it was positive. It's evident at this point that it's positive. There was even red in the stool now. That's all bleeding."

"Was Dr. Chad notified on his service that this was occurring? Was he notified by the nurse?"

"Yes, he was. And he evaluated the patient as well. He knew about the condition. He knew about the tests. He knew on that day that Mr. Brown was bleeding."

"Had he been transfused that day?"

"Yes, and that's important too. You could see that there was only a little blip in his counts that he got from the transfusion. At that point, you have to realize that something is happening with the blood after he's transfused, and the counts are still dropping. You've got to realize that this blood is going somewhere—that he's bleeding."

"What was the standard of care required of Dr. Chad?"

"At this point, Dr. Chad returns on Saturday the twenty-ninth and knows that Mr. Brown is having dark stools, and a lot of them. The patient has been tested and is positive for bleeding. Here is a patient with a significant drop in blood counts. It's urgent that you call the GI doctor to come right away and talk about getting the endoscopy done because he's in a life-threatening situation. You can't say you'll wait until the next day.

"Now what happened was Dr. Chad did call the GI doctor, but he didn't tell him to come right away. He just said Mr. Brown needed a consultation. There is no communication that the situation is urgent. The GI doctor didn't come until the following day, on Sunday the thirtieth, because that's the information he was working with."

"All right, doctor. Do you have an opinion whether the failure to do this endoscopy caused or contributed to the death of Thomas Brown?"

Dr. Sherry said yes.

"And what is that opinion?"

"Remember what blood does: it takes oxygen to places in your body, the most important place being the lungs, so more oxygen gets in the blood and goes to other places in the body. By the time the GI doctor gets there on Sunday, the thirtieth, Mr. Brown's platelet levels are too low, and they can't do the procedure. Had he come the day before on Saturday, July 29, his platelets were high enough at that time to perform the endoscopy.

"This is important to note. The platelets were at an acceptable level on Saturday, July 29, and if Dr. Chad had requested a stat consult from the GI doctor, the endoscopy could have been performed on Saturday, July 29. But even on Sunday, July 30, the GI doctor clearly said in his deposition that he told Dr. Chad he needed the platelet count to be up for the endoscopy.

"According to the GI doctor, Dr. Chad said he'd get the patient to that level—but he didn't. Remember, this is the hospitalist who makes the decisions on what to do and when to do it. He's the quarterback. But he didn't do it. He didn't give any platelets. You wonder why somebody else didn't give him—"

Mr. Cooper objected. "Asked and answered, your honor."

"Okay," Elizabeth said, appearing to agree with the defense.

"May I rule?" the judge asked, annoyed with Elizabeth. "Sustained."

Elizabeth continued, "I want to talk about the platelets again for just a moment. You believe that the failure to give platelets by Dr. Chad on Sunday, July 30 after the GI consult was a deviation from the standard of care?"

"Yes."

"Do you believe it caused or contributed to Mr. Brown's death?"

"Yes."

"Do you believe that with the endoscopy, if it had been performed on Sunday, July 30, the bleed would have been discovered and treated?"

"Yes. They would have done the procedure. They would have followed the bleeding source and adapted."

Elizabeth went on to ask Dr. Sherry three or four different ways whether or not Thomas would have lived had he had the endoscopy, and each time he said yes. She displayed on the screen the note from the GI doctor to Dr. Chad indicating that Thomas would need to be stabilized—meaning his platelet count needed to be up—in order to perform the procedure.

And he simply did not do it. It was there, plain as day for the jury to see. But Elizabeth was not done.

"Doctor, do you have an opinion as to what happened to make these platelet counts fall on the first couple of days upon entering the hospital and then continue?"

"Yes. Mr. Brown entered the hospital with a platelet count of 191."

"And when you say 191, you mean thousands, right?" Elizabeth asked.

Dr. Sherry responded, "Yes, 191,000 was Mr. Brown's platelet count when he came to the hospital. Platelets fall because when a patient gets a virus, the virus blocks the bone marrow from making platelets. For a period of time, they went down because, remember, Mr. Brown had RSV. Now, as you fight off the RSV, it goes away, and the bone marrow starts working again."

"So, what caused the levels to go down again?"

"This is what's interesting. What caused it to go down the second time was not the virus—it was the bleeding. When bleeding, the body tries to make blood clots. To do that, it's going to use platelets. That's why you need platelets. But if you're bleeding and bleeding and bleeding, your body is using up those platelets constantly trying to form those blood clots."

"And doctor, was there any recommendation by any specialist at any time that, if there was bleeding, to give platelets?"

"Yes. A hematology specialist got involved on Tuesday, July 25 because Mr. Brown's platelets were beginning to fall, and that doctor said to watch for any bleeding because they were falling. He also said, if they continue to fall, to give the patient platelets."

Elizabeth put the order from the hematologist up on the screen. "And when you get an order to monitor bleeding, do you just monitor for that day?"

"No, you don't monitor just for that day. It means to continue monitoring. You keep looking for bleeding every day."

Elizabeth continued her questioning. She and Dr. Sherry discussed discrepancies in Thomas's temperature in the records, specifically how at one point it was recorded at 104 degrees, when all other measures were just over 100. Dr. Sherry stated this must have been an error, as Thomas's temperature was taken thirty minutes after the 104 reading and it measured 100.4. So, the 104 reading was written down incorrectly. This entire line of questioning, Elizabeth told me later, was designed to knock down the defense's argument that Thomas died of an infection.

To that end, Dr. Sherry discussed Thomas's heart rate and blood pressure. He stated that if someone dies of an infection, they will always have low blood pressure. Thomas's blood pressure was normal throughout his stay in the hospital, all the way up to his passing.

It was the one thing I remembered clearly during that traumatic time—that Dr. Chad was telling me how poorly Thomas was doing, yet his blood pressure was always normal on the monitor, his heart rate always strong. It never made sense.

Dr. Sherry reiterated that everything that Thomas presented with pointed to bleeding in the stomach. It was not sepsis. It was not an infection throughout the body. It was not multisystem organ failure. Everything that happened to Thomas was a result of the GI bleed.

"Doctor, can you explain what happened to the kidneys?" Elizabeth asked.

"Yes. He had kidney failure, and he had it because the kidney specialist said it was due to the antibiotics and medicines he received."

"Are you aware from reviewing the testimony of what medicines were having this effect?"

Dr. Sherry named the antibiotics and the contrast needed for the CT scan. "Every day, the kidney specialist is making it clear on the record that his kidney issues are due to antibiotics and drugs. One can try to confuse this and say, well, the infection led to the kidney problem and that's an organ that's failing. That's not what's happening here. The kidney did not fail due to infection; it failed due to medication. The kidney specialist wrote in his notes a failure due to the antibiotics, medications, and contrast. This organ failure was not due to infection."

Elizabeth then questioned Dr. Sherry about Thomas's previous health and preexisting conditions that he had reviewed in the medical records from Everett. She ran down the list, asking Dr. Sherry if any of them in any way contributed to his death. The diabetes, the smoking twenty years prior, his stents, prior cancer—none of them, in Dr. Sherry's expert opinion, had any involvement in Thomas's death.

"I'd like to talk for just a moment," Elizabeth said, "about the recommendation that was made to place Mr. Brown in hospice. Do you have an opinion about the appropriateness of this recommendation that was made to Mrs. Brown on Tuesday morning, August 1 around 10:00 a.m.?"

"It was not appropriate," said Dr. Sherry.

Hearing him say that was heartbreaking.

Elizabeth continued, "And can you explain to the jury why this was not appropriate?"

"It was not appropriate because they said he had multisystem organ failure and he had an infection throughout his body, yet none of the evidence supported multisystem organ failure or an infection. As we talked about with the RSV, the infectious disease doctors themselves stopped the antibiotics, which they should have done.

"Dr. Chad told Mrs. Brown that her husband was in this multisystem organ failure because of an overwhelming infection, and they weren't going to be able to do anything for him. In reality, the problem was he had a very low blood count. He was bleeding, and they did not fix the bleed, which they could have done. So, they took a few things in the record, like the kidney failure, a high temp here and there, and this notion that he perhaps had the flu when he came in, and now he's dying. They tell her there's nothing they can do.

"At this point, Mrs. Brown had to make the decision whether or not she'd let him suffer because she's been told there's nothing to be done to help him. She got that advice, and she did what—"

"Objection, your honor."

"—she did what she had to do," Dr. Sherry finished.

"May I approach?" Mr. Cooper said.

"No," the judge answered. "What is your objection?"

"I'd like to approach, your honor."

"No. What is the legal basis for your objection?"

"The witness is not giving the court a medical opinion."

"New opinion," the judge said.

"It is *not* a new opinion," Elizabeth said. I smiled at how feisty Elizabeth could be.

"Do *not* speak," the judge said to Elizabeth. Frustrated, the judge motioned for them both to approach the bench. They had an inaudible conversation back and forth. Finally, as the two counsels left the bench, the judge informed the jury that Elizabeth's question was withdrawn.

Elizabeth began again with her questioning. "In the last two days of Mr. Brown's life, he was trying to go to Everett. This much is clear. They were waiting for an available ICU bed and that was the plan up until that Monday. I want to ask you—what changes did you see medically between the last day of July and the first day of August that caused this patient to go from a transfer candidate to Everett to a candidate for hospice?"

"His breathing changed," Dr. Sherry answered. "He had trouble breathing, and they weren't sure what was causing the trouble—and they didn't investigate to determine the cause of the problem."

"Do you have an opinion as to whether the doctor deviated from or fell below the standard of care in his response to the breathing episode?"

"Objection," the defense said. "There's a motion in limine on that topic."

The judge let out an aggravated sigh. "Would the jury step into the jury room, please?"

Everyone stood as the jury moved slowly out of the box. All the while, I watched seconds tick away on the clock, precious seconds that we could not afford to lose, seconds the judge was always quick to remind us we could not get back should this trial run past the end of the week.

Once again, it was decided that Elizabeth was to withdraw the question and rephrase. The judge called the jury back into the courtroom.

"Doctor, do you have an opinion within a reasonable degree of medical probability as to whether Dr. Chad fell below the standard of care in the way he addressed or failed to address the breathing problem at 8:30 in the morning, Tuesday, the first day of August?"

Dr. Sherry said yes.

"And what is your opinion, sir?"

"When Mr. Brown was having trouble breathing that early morning, Dr. Chad did not evaluate Mr. Brown for what could be causing it. He assumed it was, once again, another organ failure. He didn't do any of the appropriate testing. He didn't do an oxygen test of his blood to see what was causing it. He didn't move him to the intensive care unit, where he could be watched more carefully. He didn't do a CAT scan, where the mucus plug that was found in the autopsy would have shown up. He didn't do breathing treatments to help open up the airways. He didn't do anything when Mr. Brown had trouble breathing that morning. He just said it was another organ that was failing."

"Do you have an opinion as to what should have been done if in fact you think he was in acute respiratory failure? Do you have an opinion as to whether or not the patient at any time during his hospitalization should have been full ICU status?"

"He needed to go to the ICU when his hemoglobin fell well below normal levels, when it was at the 6.2 level. That was as early as Saturday, July 29. He was sick and bleeding. They knew there was a risk for worse things happening. For that reason, he should have been moved to intensive care then, and certainly when he had trouble breathing on that last day. If he was in the ICU, they would have been watching him more carefully and treating him—and he didn't get any of that."

"One more thing, doctor." Elizabeth handed Dr. Sherry a document. "Are you familiar with this?" Dr. Sherry agreed that he had seen it. "This is the hospital policy for transfusion. Do you have an opinion regarding Dr. Chad's adherence or failure to adhere to this policy with regard to preparing the patient for invasive procedures?"

"This policy indicates the platelet count should be seventy-five prior to invasive procedures, and in this regard, this is a hospital policy that you're showing me."

"And do you have an opinion that he deviated from the care by failing to transfuse Mr. Brown when his platelets were below seventy-five as it relates to this policy?"

"Yes. Dr. Chad deviated from the standard of care by failing to transfuse the patient when the platelet count was below seventy-five thousand, as required by this policy."

And there it was. Again. Dr. Chad knew that was the policy. He knew he needed to give Thomas platelets, as per his own hospital's policy—and he did nothing. He ignored the rules of his own hospital.

"Your honor, this concludes my examination at this time."

With that, Elizabeth yielded to Mr. Fowler, another attorney on the defense team, to begin his cross.

* * *

Dr. Sherry had done an incredible job on the stand, as had Elizabeth in her questioning. Watching the jury, I had the sense they understood the information he had relayed. So I could not wait to hear how the defense was going to handle not one, but three instances of Dr. Chad falling below the standard of care, as Dr. Sherry had explained.

Mr. Fowler began his examination, discussing many of the same topics that Elizabeth had, but he asked them in a combative and negative manner for the purpose of casting doubt on Dr. Sherry's statements. He then went into a line of questioning about a weight gain Thomas experienced in the hospital, insinuating that the anemia and the hemoglobin drop was due to this fifty-pound weight gain. Dr. Sherry disagreed, saying that a person could not possibly be given enough fluids in that time frame to cause that much gain; he believed the weight measurements were in error.

Unsatisfied, Mr. Fowler questioned Dr. Sherry on the subject in several different ways, but Dr. Sherry was unwavering. He would not change his position that any weight gain would ever affect Thomas's blood levels.

A great deal of time was spent talking about Thomas's bleed. Was it a swift bleed, a slow bleed, an oozing bleed? It appeared Mr. Fowler was trying to confuse the jury with a level of detail that did not seem to serve any purpose since the hematologist clearly said to monitor for any bleeding.

It also appeared that Mr. Fowler was not pleased with Dr. Sherry's responses, so his tone became even more sarcastic. "Let's see what else we can agree on," he said, as if Dr. Sherry had agreed with *any* of the previous discussions.

Mr. Fowler asked Dr. Sherry repeatedly about viral infections and RSV, about fevers and sepsis. Elizabeth objected on the grounds of being argumentative, which was overruled. Dr. Sherry stated again that he disagreed that RSV was the cause of death because RSV does not cause death unless a patient is immunocompromised. He repeated his assertion that there was no evidence that RSV was Thomas's cause of death.

The judge called for a bathroom break, as requested by one of the jurors. In the hallway outside of the courtroom, I saw Dr. Sherry across the way. He was pacing; it was clear he was agitated. I walked up to him and introduced myself. Tears rolled down my face in an instant.

"Thank you for everything you're doing to help us," I said. "I was so worried about whether or not what happened to Thomas could be explained in a manner that a jury could understand. You've done such a great job of doing just that."

Dr. Sherry pulled me in for a hug, and I returned it.

"Your husband never should have died," he said, his eyes moist. At that moment, we were called back. I looked up at the doctor, trying to smile, then wiped away my tears and followed him back into the courtroom.

Mr. Fowler continued with his idea that the drop in hemoglobin was due to a fluid shift and not blood loss—that there was dilution that could change the blood count. Dr. Sherry was resolute and debunked every one of Mr. Fowler's assertions. It was clear the jurors were getting restless listening to Mr. Fowler and Dr. Sherry go back and forth in disagreement.

Mr. Fowler then went on to discuss Dr. Sherry's fees for time spent reviewing medical records, reading depositions, and preparing for trial. The defense implied that there was something dark or sinister about the fact that he charged customary fees for these types of services. Elizabeth made the case later in redirect that Dr. Sherry's fees were reasonable and customary for the profession, and that in fact every other expert witness in this case charged more than Dr. Sherry.

The judge then asked the jury if they had questions for Dr. Sherry. They did not, so that concluded his testimony.

Elizabeth then called my son, Michael, to the stand.

* * *

Elizabeth began Michael's testimony by asking him questions about his presence in town for the family reunion and how he and his family stayed for almost another week to support me while Thomas remained in the hospital. Michael told the jury how he visited Thomas in the hospital, but then left with his family on Saturday, July 29 to return home to Houston, as he had to return to work that Monday. He related how he was shocked when I called him on Tuesday, August 1 about the recommendation for hospice.

Michael also testified that I was very disturbed about the quality of care provided, including the failure to consult with Thomas's primary care physician in Atlanta and the refusal to initiate the call for the doctor-to-doctor transfer. He told the jury that I was not intellectually respected by the doctors there, and while the defense asked a few questions of Michael, there was nothing in his testimony to contest.

Michael had to leave the next day, Saturday, to return home. His wife, Marna, was scheduled to fly in that Sunday evening to give her testimony on Monday. With three boys at home, they had to stagger their schedules to appear in court. I truly appreciated their efforts to do whatever was necessary to support me in this lawsuit.

After Michael left the courtroom, the judge spoke to the jury, reminding them that over the weekend they must not talk to anyone about the case or watch anything that might appear on television. They were also not permitted to google anything pertaining to the case. All of their questions had to be addressed in the courtroom, emphasizing that they must adhere to these rules to avoid a mistrial. The judge then dismissed us all for the weekend.

CHAPTER 19

THAT'S THE WAY
WE DO THINGS

ELIZABETH SEEMED CONFIDENT ABOUT THE CASE AND OUR STAR witness, Dr. Sherry. Admittedly, I felt good about his testimony too. Dr. Sherry had carefully explained Thomas's condition as it progressed each day, the actions the doctors should have considered based on Thomas's presentations, and what the doctors did and did not do, based on standard medical protocols for the medical profession. His criticisms of Dr. Chad's and Dr. Hamilton's treatments—or lack thereof—seemed sound. Dr. Sherry made it clear that they did not give Thomas the proper attention or higher level of care that he needed.

I believed that Dr. Chad and the hospital were responsible for Thomas's needless death because of the arbitrary rule that a patient must be intubated in order to be admitted to ICU. That rule did not allow any exceptions for someone in Thomas's condition. Most reprehensible was the fact that Dr. Chad lied to me when he recommended hospice for Thomas.

Dr. Chad took the fact that Thomas's kidneys were failing and turned it into this multi-organ failure narrative that simply was not true. He did not even write multi-organ failure in Thomas's chart because he knew it was false. He did not dare document that in Thomas's medical files. He even went so far as to tell me that my husband was suffering and that we should not allow him to suffer any longer. He lied about all of this to convince me to agree to send Thomas to hospice. Thomas may have been suffering, but it was due to not being treated at all until he finally died.

Why would a doctor send someone to hospice if it was not medically warranted? What was he thinking to make him believe it would be okay to tell me this? Did he really think he could lie to me and that would be the end of it? That this Black woman would just accept what had happened and go home to Georgia to bury her husband? He should have been doing *everything* he could to save Baby's life—put him in ICU and give him the platelets he needed so he could have the endoscopy to stop the bleeding.

How did this happen? How was I fooled by Dr. Chad?

Those questions were all I could think about going into that weekend—that Dr. Chad deceived me, and I agreed to let Thomas die unnecessarily. I will *never* get over this.

* * *

My sister, Tommie, my friend, Martha, whose nickname is Cookie, and I spent that weekend together, hanging out in the hotel suite watching movies and eating at various restaurants. During one of our many conversations, Tommie shared a story about an incident in 2015 at a grocery store in her neighborhood. She was shopping in the store when her friend, Maria, a baker, called her over to talk. Maria seemed very upset, and Tommie asked her what was wrong.

Prior to COVID-19, the store offered fresh-baked cookies to the children who came into the store, but the bakery manager gave instructions to not give the Black children any cookies. Maria was visibly shaken and distressed, after receiving this work directive to treat innocent Black children differently. Tommie was angry and wanted to make a formal complaint with the store manager, but Maria swore her to secrecy so she would not have any problems with the bakery manager.

Given the situation, all Tommie could do was to try to console and sympathize with Maria. "What's it to him," Tommie told Cookie and me, referring to the bakery manager. "This is not his business enterprise, his store, or his cookies." But we all knew that it was just another instance of the daily discrimination that Black people face.

During that weekend, Tommie and Cookie also tried to cheer me up, but I remained despondent, feeling partly responsible for Thomas's death. We were all very nervous about our upcoming testimonies, and it was difficult to enjoy our food. I cried myself to sleep Friday night, like I have done on so many nights.

On Saturday, November 16, Elizabeth invited us to her house to put us at ease about our testimonies. She told Tommie and Cookie to speak from their hearts about Thomas's and my relationship and what his loss had done to me. While we enjoyed our time with Elizabeth in her home, none of us felt any better about the testimonies we had to give.

I tried to prepare myself for my testimony the night before we anticipated I would be called, including carefully selecting my clothes, but the date and time for me to testify kept changing. All this uncertainty made me a nervous wreck.

* * *

On Monday morning, November 18, like clockwork, the judge reminded everyone that she was worried about the time remaining to complete the trial. She even threatened that there would be a mistrial due to us being unable to finish by that upcoming Friday. She again said that she was assigned to a case in criminal court on Monday, November 25, so there was no opportunity to schedule our case for another day—not to mention that the week of November 25 was also the Thanksgiving holiday week. The announcements continued to produce a high level of stress for just about everyone in the courtroom.

Elizabeth called our next expert witness, Dr. Alan Duffy from Everett University. She asked him about his qualifications, education, experience, and specialty in transfusion and coagulation medicine. Just as she had done with Dr. Sherry, Elizabeth asked him if he had an opinion as to why Thomas died and the cause of his death within a reasonable degree of medical probability. She also asked if he believed Thomas's death was preventable.

His answer to all these questions was a resounding yes.

Dr. Duffy indicated from the autopsy that Thomas's bone marrow was normal and working quite well. He was making new platelets and had some immature red blood cells in his bloodstream, markers for the fact that his marrow was working as hard as it could to keep up with the blood he was losing in his gut.

Under Elizabeth's questioning, he corroborated Dr. Sherry's testimony that Thomas could have been saved at any point by the endoscopic procedure to stop the bleeding. He also reaffirmed that Thomas's age and past medical history in no way contributed to his death, and that there was no multisystem organ failure.

At that, Elizabeth concluded her questioning and deferred to the defense. Mr. Cooper stepped forward for his cross-examination. His strategy was curious, because in essence, he simply repeated Elizabeth's questions and asked Dr. Duffy if he believed his answers to be correct. It seemed to me it was not helping his case because he was getting him to repeat all of Elizabeth's well-formulated points—but he had not yet shown his hand.

Mr. Cooper went after Dr. Duffy's credentials, questioning him about his expert witness work and his fellowship training. Dr. Duffy was not board-certified as a hematologist and Mr. Cooper homed in on that fact. Then, as his colleague Mr. Fowler had done with Mr. Sherry, he went after Dr. Duffy regarding his fees for appearing in court, using the same combative and accusatory tone. It was clear to me their mission was not only to discredit our experts, but to agitate them to the extent that they'd get frustrated and slip up on the stand.

Mr. Cooper's questions covered a variety of topics, from billing to Thomas's medication, then back to billing, then to RSV and the cultures done by the doctor who performed the autopsy. Then he went back to billing, at which point Elizabeth objected but was overruled.

Finally, Mr. Cooper asked Dr. Duffy, in what I found to be a badgering manner, to name each state and country where he had performed medical malpractice testimonies. Dr. Duffy was able to name several but said that he would have to refer to his records to provide a complete answer.

When Mr. Cooper was done with his questioning, Elizabeth stood for her redirect.

"Dr. Duffy, have any of your opinions been disqualified by any court of law in the United States of America or in Australia, where you have testified?"

"No, not to my knowledge."

Elizabeth looked to the defense and then to the jury, as if to signal that the defense questioning should not be taken seriously. Elizabeth then had Dr. Duffy reiterate his findings and opinions about the cause of Thomas's death, leaving that impression—not the defense's attack—in the minds of the jurors. I wanted to applaud.

* * *

Elizabeth called several other expert witnesses to the stand, asking questions similar to the ones asked of Dr. Sherry and Dr. Duffy. They all responded the same—that Thomas's bleed should have been repaired and that he could have lived.

During a break in the trial, I was introduced to Dr. Tate, an infectious disease specialist from Utah. Dr. Tate told me that he seldom comes to court as an expert witness, but every now and then, he is compelled to give his opinion in hopes of improving patient care. He went on to say that the neglect was so egregious in Thomas's case that he had to appear to help in any way he could.

I thanked him, barely able to speak. I could feel the tears welling up in my eyes, so I did not say much in an effort to hold them back.

* * *

Michael's wife Marna was next on the stand. Like Michael, she testified about how upset I was about Thomas's declining condition and how I did not understand what was happening with his care. She also spoke about how she called her father, an orthopedic surgeon, so I could speak with him for advice. She shared in Michael's shock that Thomas had been recommended to hospice after they had returned to Houston. Once again, the defense asked her a few questions, but did not contest any portion of her testimony.

We broke for lunch, at which point Elizabeth told me that Dr. Armstrong, the physician who performed Thomas's autopsy, would be testifying when we returned. She thought it best that I not sit through his testimony, as she felt it would be difficult for me to hear the description of the autopsy process and his findings. She would tell the judge that I would not be present. As reluctant as I was to miss any of the trial, I knew in my heart that she was right.

I later learned from Elizabeth that the testimony went well. She showcased Dr. Armstrong's education, extensive medical experience, and his board certification in anatomic, clinical, and forensic pathology. The physician then confirmed Thomas's cause of death as acute pulmonary edema complicated by active upper gastrointestinal hemorrhage resulting from a duodenal ulcer. Elizabeth again went through the list of Thomas's preexisting conditions and asked if they contributed to Thomas's death. Dr. Armstrong said no to each one of them.

Of course, the defense went on the offensive to discredit Dr. Armstrong. Specifically, they brought up a situation where Dr. Armstrong left a job in Georgia because a coroner wanted him to change the reason for a cause of death from a homicide to a suicide. Dr. Armstrong would do no such thing, and reminded the defense that coroners are elected officials—they aren't doctors—who may have their reasons for wanting a specific cause of death to be on the record.

The defense went on to bring up another instance where Dr. Armstrong left a position—and it turned out to be for almost the exact same reason. In this instance, Dr. Armstrong was asked to change the cause of death on a jail death case where medication was withheld from an inmate. Dr. Armstrong declared her death due to negligence, which was not well received—but the doctor would not change his declaration.

All of the defense's attempts to discredit only proved Dr. Armstrong to be a man of integrity. He would not lie, nor would he allow those organizations to ruin his reputation or put his license on the line.

Still, the defense continued their attempts to trip him up. They accused Dr. Armstrong of performing private autopsies on county time, which the doctor said was false. They tried to make him look incompetent by saying he had not reviewed Thomas's medical records before performing the autopsy, but Dr. Armstrong explained that doing so can bias the findings and that many notes do not make their way into the medical record the way they are supposed to, anyway. He only looked at medical records after he performed his autopsies.

Finally, the defense went to their go-to tactic of putting the doctor's billing on display, but according to Elizabeth, it was all for naught. Dr. Armstrong was simply too sharp for them.

* * *

Tuesday, November 19 came, and with it, another reminder from the judge about the time schedule. Elizabeth continued to reassure me that I should not worry, but it did not help. I had no choice but to trust in her confidence that we would get through this in time.

Elizabeth planned to call Dr. Chad to the stand next. Before she called on him, however, she played three recordings. One was a video recording of Dr. Chad's questioning during his deposition about the transfer to Everett. The other two recordings were audio recordings of calls with Everett. One was on Monday, July 31 at 10:04 a.m., when I insisted Dr. Chad call Everett after he sent me on that wild goose chase to contact Everett myself. The second audio recording was a call initiated by Everett to Dr. Chad later that evening at 7:09 p.m.

As soon as Elizabeth announced that she was calling Dr. Chad to the stand, Mr. Fowler stood up.

"Your honor, no objection, as long as it's not cumulative to the video depositions."

The judge agreed, and Elizabeth began her questioning.

"Doctor, I'm going to focus on Sunday, July 30, Monday, July 31, and Tuesday, August 1 right now for my questions. On Sunday, did Mrs. Brown communicate to you that she wanted her husband transferred to Everett?"

"Yes," Dr. Chad replied.

"Objection," Mr. Fowler said. "The whole transfer issue was covered on video."

"Please make a legal objection," the judge said.

"Cumulative," Mr. Fowler said.

"Thank you," the judge said. "Overruled."

Elizabeth repeated the question, and Dr. Chad once again said yes.

"On that day, did you tell Mrs. Brown that she couldn't do that herself? That it had to be a doctor-to-doctor transfer?"

"It's a doctor-to-doctor transfer, definitely, but we needed to get the accepting physician's name."

I wanted to stand up and object myself. At no point did Dr. Chad tell me anything about getting a doctor's name. All he told me at that time was that he would have to arrange the transfer, and then he asked me that insulting question about the transfer costing a lot of money. And, as I later found out, the transfer process began with Dr. Chad calling Nursing and Transfer Services at Everett—not a particular doctor.

"Did you yourself make any call to anyone at Everett in order to talk to a doctor and see if they could accept the patient on Sunday?"

"No, I did not make a call because we have a process. We give it to the case manager. The case manager works with the insurance companies. In the meantime, they give me the name of a doctor. So, all those things have to happen."

"Whether or not she can pay for transportation, they're not going to let her husband in until a doctor says he will accept them, isn't that correct?" Elizabeth asked.

"Yes, that's correct."

"And did you take any actions yourself to get a physician at Everett to accept Mr. Brown as a patient?"

Dr. Chad shifted in his seat. "As I said, there's a process. Once I have a name, I can start that process."

Elizabeth pressed him, but he continued to be evasive about the process. Dr. Chad emphasized how, as a courtesy, they let the doctors at the accepting hospital figure out for themselves who will be the admitting physician and how they have to wait for them to do that before beginning the transfer.

I was livid at witnessing his passivity and inability to get things done. Thomas's life was at stake. Should he not, as the *doctor*, just call to make a *doctor-to-doctor* transfer, so he can pass on initial medical information, like he did when I forced him to call Everett? I made a call to Everett Primary Care, and I was directed to the appropriate department in a matter of minutes. Did he not know that Everett is a highly sophisticated and efficient operation that would be able to appropriately handle his call? It was clear to me that Dr. Chad was not a proactive, assertive person that can make things happen; now he was stalling, trying to find a way around this truth.

Elizabeth turned to the jury and looked at them for a few moments as if to signal that they should take note of what was just said. Then she moved on to Sunday afternoon, July 30, when the kidney specialist came in to see Thomas.

"Mrs. Brown told him that she planned to move Mr. Brown to Everett. This is also when Mr. Brown had these dark, tarry stools. The kidney specialist writes in his notes that Mrs. Brown has talked to him about that transfer. Did you make any notation of that request?"

"No, I didn't make a note."

"But it happened, right?"

"Yes, it happened."

"And the next day, do you recall when Mrs. Brown came in that morning talking about the subject of transferring her husband to Everett?"

Dr. Chad said yes.

"Did she ask you, doctor, if you got the doctor-to-doctor transfer done? Do you recall her asking you?"

"I don't recall that question."

"Do you recall telling her it was *her* duty to get the doctor-to-doctor transfer?"

"No. I did not say that."

"Okay," Elizabeth said. "Did she bring you a piece of paper with a phone number asking you to call that number and that she would listen while you made the call? Do you remember *that*?"

"I don't recall if she handed me a paper, but, yes, we did make the transfer call. We made the call together."

How could we have made the call together if I had not attempted to first make the call myself, based on his instruction, and given him a phone number? That's how I got the direct phone number to Nursing and Transfer Services. He made that call with me at the time without regard to process. This process discussion in court was clearly nothing but a smoke screen.

"And did you speak to anyone at Everett to help get her husband transferred?"

"Again, there's a process. Our case manager was already working on it."

Over and over again, Dr. Chad deferred to their "process." In my opinion, he did not do all that he could to save a life as he waited for the process to work, despite the fact that Thomas was in dire straits. There was never any urgency in what Dr. Chad did. This was another example of a hospital rule or process dictating how a situation was handled, rather than the doctor using his better judgment to do what was in the best interest of the patient. The other example was Thomas never receiving ICU-level care for his bleeding because he did not meet some arbitrary criteria requiring intubation. So, even if the outcome meant Thomas would bleed to death while under his care, Dr. Chad was okay with that because he followed a rule.

A rule is one thing, but Dr. Chad should have exercised the appropriate judgment dependent on the circumstances and asserted himself when needed. But he never felt that need. Elizabeth drove the point home that Dr. Chad stuck with processes even when another action that was an exception to the process could have saved Thomas's life.

"Have you had a chance to listen to the transfer calls to verify your voice and the transcripts so that they're accurate?" Elizabeth asked.

Dr. Chad said he did, but Elizabeth informed me ahead of time that she knew for a fact he had not.

"During those phone calls, which we'll hear later on, did you ever express or use the term multisystem organ dysfunction or multi-organ failure when you were talking to the Everett doctors?"

"I don't remember if I used that exact term, but I did say that there were different organs that were failing."

I had taken handwritten notes during that call to Everett that I forced him to make because I knew how important that call was. He *never* said that. Elizabeth knew that too.

She then shifted to questioning Dr. Chad about the clinical resume, which is the last summary that is written up after a patient leaves the hospital. He responded that he normally only makes notes in the records once a day, despite the fact that he makes several rounds per day.

Even on the morning that he told me Thomas needed to go to hospice, he had not put those notes in the file at the time it occurred. He did not make notes of the so-called multi-organ failure. He also had not made a note that I wanted to transfer Thomas to Everett.

But then Dr. Chad went on to say that the way the doctors communicate with each other is *by their notes*.

"I want to talk about Monday now, July 31," Elizabeth continued. "You spoke to Everett on Monday, correct?"

He said yes.

"And as far as the patient's condition on Monday, there was no reason that you could think of to tell anyone that he couldn't be transferred as soon as they had a bed and said that he could go. Is that correct?"

Again, Dr. Chad said yes.

"When you came in on Tuesday, August 1, you got there before Mrs. Brown and her sister, correct?"

Again, yes.

"When you came in, did you perform a physical exam of this patient? Did you listen to his heart? Did you listen to his lungs? Did you listen to his chest? Did you do a physical exam?"

"Yes, I did all of that at the time."

"And when you did that, did you write it down in the records, in the computer, the real results of that physical exam?"

"It depends, because we only do one note a day, so after everything that happened that day is when I would make the note."

"I'm talking about a physical exam, doctor. All the systems you said were shutting down—did you make any notes in the records about the systems?"

"No, we don't put it in the clinical resume. And that day, it was a long day for us, you know?"

Elizabeth was obviously irritated. "Doctor, my question is very clear. When you came in that morning, did Mr. Brown have a change in his oxygen system?" Dr. Chad confirmed that he did. "And he was going to be transferred the last time you saw him, out to Everett, right?" He concurred. "So, at this moment in time, when you came in, he had a change in his oxygen system. Is this the event by which you recommended that he be sent to hospice?"

"Yes."

"So, you performed a physical exam. You listened to his lungs. You listened to his heart. You visually inspected his body. You touched him. But there is no record of this examination in the chart."

"Objection," Mr. Fowler said. "Argumentative."

"Overruled."

"Doctor?" Elizabeth said.

"We only do one note per day," Dr. Chad responded.

"So, if you only do one note per day, is there some rule that you can't write down the results of the physical exam in your notes?"

"That's not something we do."

"Well, if someone were going to come after you the next day and look at what you saw in terms of physical findings and an exam and it's not in your clinical resume, where would they find it?"

"Then I do a progress note."

"Where is your note? If you didn't put it in the clinical resume and you're waiting for other notes to be put in there and someone's coming behind you for whatever reason, there's no note, is that correct?"

Dr. Chad answered with a look and tone that could not have been more blasé. "That's the way we do things."

Elizabeth walked toward the witness stand. "This was the last physical exam you ever performed in Mr. Brown's life. Wasn't it important for you to document how he was doing when you did this physical?"

"Of course, it's important."

"So, what did you do with it? Did you record it? Somewhere?"

"No, because we already had the clinical resume. That was my plan for the patient for the day."

Elizabeth tilted her head and paused, indicating to the jury that this was confusing. She then continued to press Dr. Chad about the breathing complications and the examination performed by the respiratory therapist. She asked him why, when they noted his difficulties breathing, he did not see the need to move him to a higher level of care. Again, he fell back on the intubation requirement.

Then, suddenly, the judge called both attorneys to the bench. They spoke in hushed tones, too quiet for me to hear. The judge then announced a brief recess. When Elizabeth returned to our table, I could see the troubled look on her face.

Apparently, I was shaking my head at the nonsensical answers Dr. Chad had been giving, and I did not realize what I was doing. The judge told Elizabeth it was obvious that the witness was upsetting me and that she could not have me reacting in the way I was, as it might sway the jury. The judge asked Elizabeth to have a word with me during the recess.

"Dear," she said, "you can't make any show of emotions or anything—at all. You just have to sit here and listen."

"I know," I said, "but he's lying, and it's difficult to watch him lie. I didn't even know I was shaking my head. I'll do better. I promise."

After the short recess, we returned to the court, and Elizabeth resumed her examination.

"Dr. Chad, when you talked to Mrs. Brown recommending hospice, did you tell her in the conversation that you had called a pulmonary specialist, a lung doctor, to see her husband? Did you give her that piece of information?"

He shifted again in his seat. "Well, we discussed putting a scope in the patient, things like that, which is the treatment."

Another lie. Dr. Chad did not tell me anything of the sort at that moment. When I walked in there that morning, Mable, the nurse, told me that Thomas's blood was "really bad," and Dr. Chad told me that all his organs were failing. He told me that we needed to make Thomas comfortable so that he did not suffer.

Elizabeth asked again, "Did you tell her that you had called for a specialist?"

Dr. Chad finally stopped evading and answered, "No. I did not say that."

"Did you tell Mrs. Brown in any words that there was nothing more that could be done for him and that he would need to be kept comfortable?"

"That is correct."

"And how long did it take for the entire encounter between you and Mrs. Brown? Can you tell me?"

"I would say forty-five minutes."

Lies upon lies upon lies. That conversation lasted five minutes, if even that long. Elizabeth asked him again, because she knew from our previous conversations that the discussion was far shorter, yet he reiterated that he spoke to me for close to an hour.

Elizabeth then shifted her questioning. "What's the level of platelets a patient must have for an invasive procedure?"

"I just learned that it's about seventy-five thousand," Dr. Chad responded.

Just learned?

Elizabeth pressed on. "So, if the patient needs to have platelets, you can order them, right? But you just didn't think, in this case, that you needed to do that?"

"There was no order for an endoscopy because the patient was too unstable for various reasons. The patient had sepsis and renal failure. He was on dialysis. He had encephalopathy. His brain was failing, and his lungs were failing. His bone marrow was failing as well, and he had a blood clot in his arm. A patient can die for all of these reasons."

"So, when the GI doctor had in his notes that the patient was unstable for an endoscopy, you expected the GI doctor to tell you to give platelets? Did you know that the platelets were low?"

"Yes, I knew that they were low."

"Are you saying that the GI doctor has to tell you that this patient, who needs an endoscopy and has low platelets, needs platelets? You, as his primary treating physician, don't *you* have the *responsibility* to give him some platelets so that he can do the endoscopy and stop the bleeding?"

"Whenever the doctor is ready to order the endoscopy, then we order the platelets. They only last twelve to twenty-four hours. I have to know when the endoscopy is going to be scheduled so I know when to order the platelets."

Dr. Chad's answer clearly pointed out the complete lack of communication between all the doctors involved in Thomas's care. No one cared enough to take the next step to confirm who would give Thomas the platelets and when the surgery would occur, so nothing happened for days.

"Are you as a hospitalist in charge of the patient's care?" Elizabeth asked with intensity in her tone.

"No. All of us are in charge of this patient's care. It's a team effort. It's not just me."

"Well, who's leading the team, doctor?" she demanded, satisfied that she had Dr. Chad in the position of answering difficult questions that got to the heart of the matter. "Who's the person? Who's the primary care physician?"

"I am the attending doctor."

"So, do you have a job? Do you as a primary care doctor have the job to find out what any specialist you call in wants done? Or does everybody do what they want?"

"I put the orders in. Everybody does their own thing, and I make sure that everything they do isn't in conflict with each other. I coordinate the care plan. That's what I do. They all do their own thing."

"When you call in different doctors, do you coordinate the care? They don't have to talk to each other?"

"We talk to each other through the chart."

But the chart isn't updated during the day, only at the end of the day.

Elizabeth was unrelenting in her pressure. Over and over, she asked Dr. Chad if he was responsible for everything, and he kept deferring to the notion that patient care was everyone's job. They were a team. They all worked together—which was code for "not my responsibility."

Elizabeth continued to push him until he just came right out and shouted, "Mr. Brown needed to die with dignity!"

I was shocked, and I know it showed on my face. This was the first time I had heard that said.

It was not up to Dr. Chad to decide what was dignity and what was not. It was *my* decision, and as Thomas's wife, I needed to be given all the information so that I could make an informed decision about Thomas's care. Had I been given the complete information, I know I would have said that I wanted to hear what the pulmonary doctor was going to say. I would have wanted Thomas to get the highest level of care in the *official* ICU. I would have wanted everything possible to be done for him. But the way Dr. Chad presented it to me, there were no other options except hospice, and all I knew was I could not let Thomas suffer.

Elizabeth went back to pressuring Dr. Chad about the ICU and why Thomas was not moved there. She was trying to make him nervous, to get him to say something more outrageous than he already had. He even went so far to say that the pulmonary tests would require some type of tool similar to an endoscope to examine his lungs, and that he presented that option to me.

I could not believe it. Earlier, he had evaded the question when asked if he told me about the pulmonary consult because he had not.

Then, Dr. Chad had the unmitigated gall to say that the family told him that the best course of action, based on Thomas's wishes, was to send him to hospice. He did not want to be a burden to us. He did not want to be bedbound or in a wheelchair. He did not want to be connected to tubes or a mechanical ventilator.

We didn't tell him that the best course of action was hospice! Who am I to decide what is the best course of action medically? He recommended hospice—even when there were other courses of actions to be taken to save his life!

Dr. Chad took what I shared about my husband's wishes and twisted it to misrepresent the truth. He also left out the important fact that I told him that Thomas and I wanted everything possible to be done to save Thomas's life. *What is wrong with this man's thinking? His judgment?*

It should have been very simple: do everything they could for Thomas. They—Dr. Zeller or Dr. Chad—should not have guessed beforehand about outcomes when there were options still available to get Thomas through his sickness. But they were indifferent. Saving Thomas's life was not a priority.

Elizabeth continued to press Dr. Chad. "So, did you tell Mrs. Brown that there was absolutely no positive thing you could do while her husband was not on a breathing tube? None of those things, like multi-organ shutdown or nonfunctioning bone marrow, were happening to him while you were having this conversation, were they?"

Dr. Chad could not help but show his lack of judgment again.

"No. I'm explaining what's going to happen in the future if we proceed with the pulmonology consult. And endoscopy is not without risks, okay? The risk could outweigh the benefits. People die when they do the endoscopy. Look at Joan Rivers. She passed away on the endoscopy table."

"Dr. Chad, you talk about the risk of an endoscopy—Joan Rivers died of medical negligence. You do know that, don't you, by the way? You do know that, right?

"Yes."

Wow! Did he just use an example of medical negligence to support his position?

"Okay. So, let's just keep on this case. Okay?"

It was clear Elizabeth sensed Dr. Chad's distress, and she pressed on. "Did you say that you believed that the risk of endoscopy was greater than the risk that he might die if he didn't have an endoscopy? Is that what you just said?

"Yes."

"Okay. Could he possibly have a worse result than he did when he was taken off dialysis, taken off blood transfusions, and sent to hospice, where he had no further support? Could he possibly have come out any worse, if he'd had an endoscopy?"

"If Mr. Brown did not go to hospice, what would have happened was that he would have eventually tired out with his breathing. They were going to put a tube in his throat, put him in a mechanical ventilator, and put a tube in his belly for feedings. And eventually, I think—I *believe*—that he would eventually pass away with all of those things that are unnecessary. He needed to die with dignity. He died in hospice with dignity."

"When did you make that decision, doctor? Because you arranged the transfer to Everett the day before."

"It was the first. August 1."

"And that's when you decided that this was the best course for Mr. Brown?"

"Yes."

"Doctor, you could have ordered a CT scan that could have found the mucus plug. They could have sucked it out, and perhaps he wouldn't have had a respiratory arrest. Did you order a CT scan?"

"No, I did not."

"Last question. Doctor, is it your job to determine what dying with dignity looks like for Mrs. Brown, once she is fully advised of all of the options?"

"I would say there's an ethical obligation for physicians to discuss both options to the family, and dying with dignity is one of the best options that we could offer to the family, rather than letting Mr. Brown suffer through all of those things unnecessarily. It would not change the outcome."

"Okay. I have nothing further," Elizabeth said.

Mr. Fowler said, "Same. We'll reserve, your honor."

I tried to remain expressionless during Dr. Chad's testimony, putting all of my energy into my clenched hands. It was a relief when it was over, and I asked myself how much more of the lies and twisting of the truth I had to listen to in this courtroom while being expected to show no emotion.

The answer was: it did not matter. There were others yet to take the stand—including me.

CHAPTER 20

I BELIEVED HIM

THE NEXT FEW DAYS LEADING UP TO MY TIME ON THE STAND WERE a bit of a blur.

First up on Tuesday morning, November 19, a video recording was shown of the GI doctor that would have performed the endoscopy. Under Elizabeth's questioning, he stated that after his consultation with Thomas on Sunday, July 30, he discussed with Dr. Chad exactly what the situation was. When Elizabeth pressed him for specifics, he waffled, saying that he did not remember exact conversations with any physicians but that he normally will tell the lead physician whether or not a patient is stable or unstable for surgery, and what needs to be done to stabilize them.

Then Elizabeth got him to say something incredibly important. The GI doctor stated that if they had transfused Thomas and continued to transfuse him, keeping his blood counts up, he would have survived.

This statement spurred an immediate objection from Mr. Cooper. The judge told both sides to approach, and after some discussion, she overruled his objection. Elizabeth concluded her questioning on that powerful statement from the GI specialist. It was a good way to start the day.

Next on the witness stand was my friend, Cookie. She testified about how long we have been friends and how difficult it was for me during the course of the hospital stay. She also talked about how several of us friends traveled together to Las Vegas on an annual basis to celebrate birthdays. I noticed that they left the cross-examination to a younger white woman on their team, who did not contest any part of Cookie's testimony. The nastiness and trickery was reserved for the old white men.

Tommie followed Cookie's testimony, offering similar information about how long she had known Thomas. She also talked about how all of us would travel together over the years and how much fun we had, with Thomas being the life of the party and always looking after all of the women in the group. She knew him longer than I did, and to this day, she tells me how much she misses that back-and-forth banter with him.

Elizabeth then showed the video deposition of Dr. Bernard Armstrong, Thomas's primary physician at Everett. Elizabeth had come to Atlanta to interview him, and he agreed to talk about Thomas's health based on his nearly twenty-five-year medical history at Everett. He stated that Thomas was a healthy man, diligent about his healthcare, and did what his doctors recommended. His diabetes had been controlled for more than twenty years, he was only on an oral medication, never insulin, and those meds had recently been reduced due to Thomas's controlling the condition so well. Dr. Armstrong painted a truthful and vibrant picture of Thomas as a strong, healthy man.

After the video, Elizabeth called Dr. Chad to the stand for a second time. Her sole purpose was to exert more pressure on him, to catch him in more lies. She questioned him again about the discussion between himself and the GI doctor about the requirements for the endoscopy. Mr. Cooper, of course, objected, but Elizabeth retracted and rephrased. She asked Dr. Chad if he went to the other consultants to tell them why Thomas was not being scoped. Over and over, Dr. Chad stated that they communicate through the chart. With each declaration of that fact, it became crystal clear that their lack of communication played a significant role in Thomas's death.

As they went on, Dr. Chad again referred to all of the issues that he felt kept Thomas from being scoped—the fever, the sepsis, the inability to eat. Elizabeth had had enough.

"Doctor, these criteria you referred to look more like a history of his health problems, not what needs to be corrected before he can be scoped. Do you understand that these can be two different things?"

"Yes."

"Let me ask you then—did you have any idea on Monday, the thirty-first, that one of the criteria the GI doctor wanted was platelets? That the platelets were too low? Did you know that?"

"It's in there that he had pancytopenia." Pancytopenia is a deficiency in the red cells, white cells, and platelets.

"Let me ask this again, doctor. Did you know that one of the reasons that Mr. Brown would not be scoped was because his platelets were too low?"

Mr. Cooper objected, and the judge sustained the objection on the grounds that Elizabeth had already asked the question.

"Okay, doctor," Elizabeth said. "I want to give you a hypothetical. The GI doctor says he needs to perform an endoscopy so he can find this bleed, but he needs platelets up to his personal requirements. It's possible he said this to you, right?"

"He might have told me that."

"Okay. Would you not give the platelets for any reason?"

"He never indicated to me that he needed the platelets right away. There was no need to do the procedure right away. As I said, there were six other conditions we were looking at before we would get the platelets. When the patient was ready, the GI doctor would let me know if the patient fit his criteria for endoscopy, and then I would get the platelets."

Whether she was satisfied or frustrated by his answer, I could not tell, but Elizabeth thanked Dr. Chad and told him that was all she had for him. The defense crossed, primarily repeating Elizabeth's questions, but making sure to draw attention to the fact that the GI doctor's notes did not indicate that the endoscopy was urgent and therefore neither were the platelets. They also highlighted the fact that one of the other consultants stated that no transfusion was needed, despite the fact Thomas's platelets had dropped precipitously.

Hearing all this, it was apparent to me that Dr. Chad simply was lax in reading each and every note in the record. He did not gather any information that was not in the notes until the end of the day, nor did he properly analyze Thomas's condition to understand the big picture. If he had done that, he would have realized that the notes indicated one doctor did not know what the other was doing and that he needed further clarification from the GI doctor.

Instead, Dr. Chad read the words in the chart and did not perform any kind of critical analysis or interpretation. He read one note and accepted it. His judgment again appeared to be flawed in thinking that

Thomas's other medical conditions had to be resolved in order to meet the GI doctor's requirements for endoscopy. Dr. Chad was the so-called quarterback, but he seemed to be sitting back and waiting for direction from others, seldom asking questions and seeking critical information to make decisions.

All this time, I was wondering, *Why? Is this the way he treats all of his patients? Or is it just how he treats his Black patients?* Even the consultants seemed to take minimal interest in Thomas's condition. Not one of them was assertive in ensuring that Thomas's care was progressing in a satisfactory manner to save his life. If Thomas had been white, would he still be alive? Given the disparity of the delivery of healthcare to Black people in this country, it was not a stretch to think that was the case here.

In my mind, nothing else made sense.

* * *

Both Elizabeth and the defense juggled the times when their witnesses testified. Time was running short, and certain out-of-town witnesses could not change their schedules. That meant my time to testify kept getting bumped too.

The defense brought forth their witnesses on Wednesday, Thursday, and Friday. They continued to mislead the jury, as they had done in the questioning of our witnesses, distorting the truth whenever they could. One of the most shocking statements made by a defense witness was by Dr. Barber from Tampa, who testified that the platelets should be saved for those patients who are injured and are in the trauma unit.

My goodness! Saved for the trauma unit? Why was Thomas not worthy of the platelets? He had an immediate need. Why was that not equivalent to those in the trauma unit?

* * *

On Thursday, November 21, before the jury entered the courtroom, the judge again warned us of the impending deadline. She went so far as to tell both attorneys to settle this case out of the kindness of their hearts because she was concerned about finishing on time.

Of course, that did not happen.

When the jury was present, the judge explained to them that this was likely going to spill over into Monday of the next week. She then asked that each juror come back after lunch with a written note telling her whether or not they could return on Monday, November 25 to complete the case.

After lunch, the judge read each juror's note one by one. It turned out they were all able to return on Monday, and the judge announced that she was able to get her Monday case postponed to Tuesday, November 26. It was extra drama on a day when I was already anxious about my testimony, but we really did need that extra day.

Finally, on that same day, Thursday, November 21, Elizabeth called me to the witness stand.

* * *

Elizabeth had spent hours during the past year coaching me on the best way to express myself during my testimony. She also prepared me for the way in which the defense might attack me with their questions. At the same time, she told me not to worry about any of it because I had done nothing wrong; it was the hospital that had to defend their actions and explain why Thomas had died while in their care.

Still, despite preparing and dressing meticulously for the occasion, I was nervous. All eyes were on me as I walked to the stand, but I decided I was not going to look at the jury. I would only look at the person who posed questions to me and look to Elizabeth for encouragement and strength. I tried to block everyone else in the courtroom out of my mind.

Elizabeth asked me questions about how I met Thomas, how I initially was not interested in him because he was so handsome, how we called each other "Baby," and how we helped each other through college. She asked about raising our kids and traveling the country and the world with Michael as he aspired to and became an Olympian. I discussed my degrees and credentials, as well as the jobs I have held in my lifetime.

Then I told the story of how everything happened in the hospital, why I decided to get an autopsy, and how I decided to seek a lawyer to help me get to the bottom of why this entire hospital experience was so strange and went so wrong.

Elizabeth asked, "Why did you seek legal assistance immediately?"

"The entire time I was there, it was my intuition that something was wrong, that Thomas was not getting the best care. Thomas has always looked after me and protected me, and I couldn't do the same thing for him in that hospital. So this is why I'm here. I'm still fighting for him."

Elizabeth tried to anticipate everything the defense would ask me so that the jury heard it from me first, and she did an excellent job. Once Elizabeth finished her questioning, though, it was the defense's turn.

Mr. Cooper started his cross-examination with the details of my attempts to contact Thomas's primary care physician at Everett. He seemed to want to make a point of the fact that Dr. Armstrong had tried to reach me but could not—something I had not learned until I saw his video deposition. There were so many calls coming from friends and family that I simply missed the notification of his call. It was not clear to me why he was pursuing this line, but he quickly moved on.

Mr. Cooper then moved on to the speech pathologist's assessment of Thomas's inability to swallow properly. "You were upset about an order being entered for a feeding tube. If a speech pathologist evaluated him and said that she felt it was dangerous for him to try to eat or drink or even eat ice chips, why is it that you're upset about the tube feed order?"

"I was upset because of the lack of communication. I was there almost all of the time. It seemed that the feeding tube was inserted during the little time I was not at Thomas's bedside. I was always asking questions. I didn't object to him being on a feeding tube or any action that would save Thomas's life. I wanted them to talk to me and let me know what was going on. That's all I wanted. I wanted to be in control of my husband's care. I didn't want things to happen where I wasn't informed."

I could feel myself getting angry and took a breath to compose myself.

"All right," Mr. Cooper said, "so in the care coordinators' note on Sunday, July 30, it says that the patient's family would like the patient to be transferred to Everett Hospital in Georgia. She writes that Dr. Chad is trying to get a physician at Everett to accept the patient, but you say this note is incorrect?"

"*I* was the one who insisted Dr. Chad make that first call to Everett, and it appears on the recordings we heard yesterday that it was Everett following up with *him*. Therefore, Dr. Chad never initiated one call on my husband's behalf, so for that note to indicate that Dr. Chad initiated calls and made things happen is incorrect."

"It also says that the patient's family would like the patient transported via air ambulance. Given that money was going to come out of your pocket, you think it wasn't appropriate for Dr. Chad to mention that it was going to be expensive for you to pay for that yourself?"

"I just don't think he should have said that in that tone. The way he said it was insulting and demeaning, as if I couldn't possibly have that amount of money. I took it as an insult."

Mr. Cooper moved on.

"This note from Monday, July 31 states that a nurse placed a call to Everett and spoke to their transfer service. She was informed a doctor at Viewpark would need to call the transfer services line to initiate the transfer request. She was also informed she needed to talk to another department about insurance." He referenced slides up on the screen. "We see that the insurance company provided authorization for Everett to accept the patient. You realize that they had to go through this process, right?"

"Yes. The nurse approached me and told me about the insurance situation. But *I* was the one who resolved the insurance issue. I got on the phone to call BCBS myself because I didn't understand why an authorization would take two days. I selected the best insurance in the country as a federal government employee. The woman at BCBS told me that I didn't need a pre-certification—that just like we walked into Viewpark to get care, we could walk into Everett emergency and get care, or fly to Everett and get care. There was no problem with that on the insurance company's end. I'm the one who did everything on my own to try to help speed up this process. *You* said it was going to take a couple of *days*. I got it done in thirty minutes or less."

"But you understand, Mrs. Brown, that there was a process that had to be completed, that they had to go through in order to make sure that insurance would pay for him once he got to Everett."

"I just answered that." I bit my lip as soon as I said it. I knew Mr. Cooper was pressing me, asking me the same question to rile me up—and he had. I am sure he already knew how I felt about him and Mr. Fowler. My father always jokingly told me to never play poker because the look on my face always gave away my personal thoughts and feelings.

"All right," Mr. Cooper said, "so we heard the two calls with Dr. Chad and Everett, one that you were on and one that came later." I agreed. "And the one in the morning was you and him calling Everett to basically explain the situation to them."

I stopped him. "That is not correct. Dr. Chad refused to call Everett. I insisted that he make that initial call. You're incorrect in saying that he worked with me and we called Everett together. That was not how it happened."

"Okay, let's look at the 7:30 p.m. call that evening when Everett called him back. Dr. Chad said he wasn't at his computer and didn't have all the information. In your interpretation of that part of the call, Dr. Chad said that he could put the patient on a regular floor. You're criticizing him for that?"

"Yes, and here's why. Listen to the first call. Dr. Chad called off several of the conditions that Thomas was experiencing—melena, kidney injury, RSV, bronchitis, on two liters of oxygen. The Everett doctor immediately responds by asking if Thomas is in the ICU. Even they felt, after hearing this list of five or six conditions, that this was a critical situation and Thomas should be in ICU. Then on the second call, Dr. Chad must have said five times, frantically, 'He's stable, he's stable, put him on the regular floor.' This is a perfect example of the confusion and lack of clear communication at Viewpark Hospital. Dr. Chad says he's stable just so he can send my husband on his way to a floor that's not appropriate for him, while Everett knows that Thomas should be in an ICU."

As Mr. Cooper continued on this line of questioning, Elizabeth objected but was overruled. Mr. Cooper continued to try to wear me down, and to be honest, I was irritated at how deviously he twisted the truth. I worried about the jury being confused.

Mr. Cooper asked me if I saw Dr. Chad as helpful since he was trying to get Thomas on a general floor so that they could get him moved. I responded no, that I questioned Dr. Chad's judgment of putting him on a regular floor when he was seriously bleeding. On that second Everett call, Dr. Chad seemed frantic as he repeatedly told Everett that Thomas was stable enough to be put on a regular floor, but then the next morning, Dr. Chad told me there was no hope and Thomas needed to go to hospice. This just did not make sense.

Mr. Cooper quickly changed the subject, asking me about the consent to transfer Thomas to hospice. I reiterated that I was led to believe there was absolutely no hope for Thomas and that nothing could be done—that Dr. Chad told me that we needed to make him comfortable.

"I was not going to make my husband suffer," I said, my voice shaking. "I believed him. I believed the doctor."

Mr. Cooper then directed me to the chaplain's note that said the spouse said, "I'm ready. I don't want this. I'm ready for hospice."

"I never said I wanted hospice, and you are misinterpreting my words. What I meant when I said 'I don't want this'—and maybe I didn't say it very well under the circumstances—was that I didn't want this to happen to my husband. I was in shock. I didn't want my husband to die. I didn't want this situation to be. I never even thought of the word hospice until it was presented to me, so I *know* I didn't say, 'I'm ready for hospice.'"

Mr. Cooper then questioned me again about the specifics of the hospice orders. He pointed out that the hospice nurse indicated that Thomas was bedfast and required total care, such as hygiene and turning, and that I had stated that I did not want any artificial or internal feeding. Once again, I told them that I was led to believe there was no hope and that I did not want Thomas to suffer.

"But it further says that the patient's wife decided to go with hospice and will be transferred to the inpatient hospital today. Isn't that correct?"

I was so glad that Elizabeth anticipated that I would be asked about that note. "No, that's not correct. You know, you have everything kind of twisted. You said the patient's wife *decided*. I didn't decide anything. I *agreed*. There's a big difference."

"There were numerous doctors involved in taking care of your husband. Did you seek to discuss their opinion with anyone else?"

"No. I believed his doctor. He was the one in charge."

In the witness chair, I could hear the discussions before the bench, and there were moments when Elizabeth objected to Mr. Cooper's questions and told the judge that he was trying to get me to say something that would cause a mistrial. Luckily, Elizabeth had prepared me well, and it never came to that. But the effort left me drained, nonetheless.

Mr. Cooper went on to list every doctor involved in Thomas's case and whether or not I asked for their advice. Each time, I got less patient, but gave him the same answer. "I believed the doctor."

I wanted to ask Mr. Cooper if he was trying to insinuate that Dr. Chad did not make the right call, and therefore, I should not have believed him, that it was my responsibility to check up on Dr. Chad and all of the specialists for their opinions. Elizabeth had anticipated this, however, and told me not to do that. She was adamant that I only answer their questions and that on the redirect she would ask the questions to clear everything up. Even knowing that, it was all I could do to keep my mouth shut and not add additional commentary. I cannot recall a time outside of the entire hospital experience when I was more frustrated.

Mr. Cooper brought up again my discussions about Thomas's wishes regarding life-prolonging measures. Again, I corrected him on the misconstruing of those words and stated, again, that Dr. Chad made me believe there were no further options at that point.

Then the defense went in a direction I had not expected.

Mr. Cooper showed me a picture. "Did you take this photograph?" I said I had. "And this was taken in hospice? And then there's this picture of your husband after he had passed away?"

"Yes."

"Why would you take these pictures of your husband in the hospital and in the transport to hospice and in hospice and after he had passed? Didn't you see an opportunity to sue, and so you took these pictures so you would have them?"

At that moment, all I could do was stare at him. I swear I saw evil in his eyes. I blinked back tears and continued to stare. I felt like I was looking at the devil, because how else could this man stand here and accuse me of allowing my husband to die so I could sue? Frankly, I was hesitant to look at this evil man—but I would not look away. I said no and shook my head, disgusted as he kept up the pressure.

"The hospice nurse offered you a second opinion when you first got there, but you decided not to do that, right?"

I was trembling, but I answered. "She was just reading me the company line. I could tell there was no one really concerned about Thomas. By that time, the decision was made based on what Dr. Chad had told me."

"And so that night, as your husband passed away, you got on the computer and started Googling and looking for lawyers, correct?"

I said yes.

"And it was one of those lawyers who said you needed an autopsy and to call Dr. Armstrong, correct?"

I told him that I asked the attorney if he could recommend someone in the area and that it happened to be Mr. Armstrong.

"Thank you, Mrs. Brown."

The judge called for a brief recess. I stepped down from the witness stand, shaken.

During the break, I told Elizabeth that if those people at Viewpark Hospital had been kind and compassionate toward me, perhaps I could have accepted Thomas's death as an unfortunate and untimely circumstance and gone on with my life. But their callousness, like that of their attorneys, indicated to me in every respect that I needed to pursue this action.

"A good bedside manner covers a multitude of sins, says the good doctor, Peter Gulden, my deceased first husband," Elizabeth said.

* * *

When we returned to the courtroom, Elizabeth questioned me again, allowing me to clarify that I was the family historian and that I took pictures frequently of events that happened in the family, and that it was not extraordinary for me to take pictures of Thomas. I talked about the family history book that I had compiled and disseminated at the family reunion in Florida, and how I often created photo books for various holidays or celebrations. I talked about how I had created a photo book entitled "Remembering Grandpa" for our grandchildren to help them to always remember him.

Between Elizabeth and the defense, I was on the stand most of the day. I was emotionally exhausted as I struggled to follow Elizabeth's coaching and guidance, while correcting the misconceptions that the defense tried to perpetrate. I was so relieved when my testimony was over.

There was no limit to what the defense would do to win their case, including accusing me of purposely letting Thomas die, as if his care was within my control. I was frustrated because I could not respond in the way I wanted when asked a question; I had to wait until my attorney followed up. Mr. Cooper was so malicious in his questioning that it would surely leave a lasting impression with the jury. I could only hope that I had left one too.

CHAPTER 21

THE LAST CHAPTER WILL BE WRITTEN IN THIS COURTROOM

Cookie left Orlando for home the day after she completed her testimony, Wednesday, November 20. Tommie left for home on Thursday, November 21. That meant that I was now alone in Orlando, but I did not mind. I looked forward to having a quiet weekend and hanging out in the suite most of the time. I planned to watch movies, to nap whenever I felt like it, and to take care of me.

Elizabeth and I met on Sunday afternoon for lunch. I came with a list of questions for her. I knew she was fully prepared for the closing statement the following day, but I asked her to please allow me to ask my questions of her so I could put my mind at ease.

We talked about all the items on my list, but the most disturbing issue for me was that the hospital did not seem to take any responsibility for creating all of Thomas's medical issues that he had at the end; they seemed to focus on how serious his conditions were as if he came to the hospital with those conditions. Thomas was a healthy man when we came to that hospital that first day, but that point seemed to be lost in most of the testimonies.

While we were eating our lunch, Michael called me. He and his family were driving from Houston and would be in town that evening. They wanted to hear the closing arguments and the verdict, and they were coming to support me! I immediately broke down crying. I was trying to be strong, but the case had taken its toll, and I found myself unable to keep my emotions in check at almost every turn.

When I told Elizabeth that Michael was coming, a broad grin spread across her face. She already knew. She and Michael had coordinated his return.

Elizabeth constantly amazed me from the very first time I spoke with her. She was not just my attorney—she was my friend, and she truly cared. I was so fortunate to have found her.

* * *

Elizabeth gave her closing statement on Monday, November 25.

"Jurors, I want to thank you for all the time, all the note-taking, everything you have done to give your attention to this case. The system depends on you. At one o'clock, this will be in your hands, and then we all hurry up and wait to see what you come up with." There were some smiles from the jurors at that. "When we went through this process of selecting you, we all listened carefully to everything you said, and we all placed our trust in you to be fair and to be just in your determinations. And we still have that trust. All of us do. And we thank you for that.

"Let's talk about the greater weight of evidence and what we must prove. We must prove that, more likely than not, that the care of Dr. Hamilton and Dr. Chad was negligent and that it was a substantial cause of the death of Thomas Brown. That means they were not reasonably careful in their jobs as doctors, and therefore, that is a legal cause of Mr. Brown's death. Mr. Brown died because of an ulcer he developed in the hospital, which wasn't treated for a long enough period of time. Dr. Hamilton and Dr. Chad failed to timely diagnose and treat a bleeding ulcer, which was a legal cause of his death."

Elizabeth went on to summarize Thomas's journey through the hospital, from the regular floor to the progressive care unit to the unofficial ICU. She stated that he was never given the highest level of care, despite being sick enough to warrant it. In fact, they bypassed the highest level, sending him to the lowest level, which was hospice.

She restated all of the pertinent facts of the case, much like she had done in her opening statement, this time including the testimony of the two truly independent experts—the hospice doctor who put the cause of death on the death certificate and Dr. Armstrong, the physician I hired to perform the autopsy. Elizabeth pointed out that they both agreed on the GI bleed as the cause of death—two independent doctors drawing the exact same conclusion, which was prolonged bleeding without any intervention.

Elizabeth continued to recap: the phone calls with Everett, the poor communication in the medical notes—especially between the GI doctor and Dr. Chad—and how I took matters into my own hands to get Thomas the best and most appropriate care possible by trying to set up the transfer to Everett and clear the health insurance hurdle. Then she turned to the hospice conversation.

"Then Dr. Chad told Mrs. Brown her husband's organs were shutting down. He would not live. 'He only has twenty-four to forty-eight hours to live, and you need to make him comfortable. There is nothing else we can do.' She chose to do what she thought was best for him. She signed the necessary paperwork. And as we know, she was not at peace with all this and wanted to know what happened. Something didn't seem right, and she took the courageous steps to find out exactly what happened to her beloved husband—hard steps. She allowed her husband's body to go to a pathologist and be opened up—that body that had been by her side for forty-five years. It's not an easy choice—not a choice you make unless you know in your heart that you really must know what happened."

Elizabeth saying that brought tears to my eyes, and I lowered my head. She continued to list the facts as she had presented them throughout the trial, but it was hard to listen to all of that again—until she got to the question as to why Thomas had not been given platelets. I looked up because I heard a waver in her voice. Her eyes looked wet.

"Why wasn't Thomas Brown given those platelets? What were they thinking? That one unit of platelets was better used on someone else? Why wasn't Mr. Brown worthy of receiving platelets?" She took a breath and let the question settle in with the jurors. Once she composed herself, she moved into one of the most moving and heartfelt parts of her statement.

"Mr. and Mrs. Brown came to this city for a family reunion. When Mr. Brown wasn't feeling well, she took him first to urgent care and then the hospital because she just wanted to get medical care for him. She went there for help. People go to the hospital for help. He was admitted for observation, and that's what they did—they observed him to death.

"They knew what was wrong. They knew there were stress ulcers as a result of all the medications they had given him. That's not surprising at all. What is surprising, shocking, and absolutely unbelievable is that he developed a known condition that frequently results from taking antibiotics and the contrast for the CT scan—something they expected because it happens to plenty of people—and they did nothing to fix it. They discovered it in time to take care of it, and they did nothing about it. In a hospital in the United States of America, a man came in without risks and was slowly allowed to bleed to death without anybody doing anything. They talked about it. They made notes in the chart. But they did nothing.

"Mrs. Brown, since the care was not quality care, made calls right after Mr. Brown passed away and was told to get an autopsy. Without that autopsy, we would not be here today, and what happened to Mr. Brown would all be buried. No one would have known Jonnie Brown.

"She believed she had to do something to get help for her husband. She wondered why they wouldn't call Everett for his medical records. Why they wouldn't call Everett to initiate the doctor-to-doctor transfer. Imagine the tremendous anguish, the tremendous duty she felt to take care of her husband the way he always cared for her.

"Mr. Brown served in the Air Force. Went to Vietnam to serve his country and to protect us. Her son represented our country in the Olympics. She has a high-level security clearance working for the Department of Homeland Security. And she didn't want to go back home because home now is a place of enormous loneliness and sadness. She volunteered to come back to Orlando through FEMA to work long hours to help Floridians who suffered through Hurricane Irma. She did that to get her heart and head away from thinking about her home that is now without the love of her life.

"Everything in her life has changed. Simple things. Walking the dog together, meals together, and talking about their plans for the future—just enjoying each other's company. Every part of her world is completely torn, but even so, she had the courage to do everything she's done because, as she said on the stand, she is still fighting for Thomas. The last chapter of the story is going to be written in this courtroom.

"There are two questions on the verdict form. Did either of these doctors cause or contribute to, by their inaction or action, the death of Thomas Brown? If the answer is 'no,' you're done, sign it, and that's it. If you find it more likely than not that their actions were a substantial cause, then you must answer 'yes.'

"The second question asks you, based on your life experiences, based on your common sense, based on your knowledge of love and companion-ship and long-term relationships that you bring to us here, to consider Mr. Brown's role as the patriarch of the family—how they lived, how they shared all their responsibilities, in sickness and in health, the promises they made to each other, how they loved each other. How much did Jonnie Brown lose when Thomas Brown was buried in a mili-tary funeral in Los Angeles, California? Damages in this case are for mental pain and suffering. For all of those horrible days in the hospital trying to do everything she could to save him—and she failed.

"She failed him in her mind. She had to, through this courageous process, learn the bitter truth: in her quest for knowledge and justice, she learned that she signed away her husband's chances to live. She said to you that she will carry this for the rest of her life.

"It is my duty to her to give you my thoughts about what will be fair. You don't have to accept it. You may think it's not enough. You may think it's too much. It's completely your decision."

Elizabeth told the jurors the amount we sought in damages by showing her calculations, based on the time frame from the date of Thomas's death until a date representative of the average future life expectancy for men in the US. When she delivered the number, she again said that she trusted them to make the right decision and to adjust the award amount to be more or less as they deemed appropriate. She thanked them for their time and sat down.

During the nearly two years we had been working together to prepare for the case, I had never asked Elizabeth how much money I could be awarded. The amount was not of primary interest to me because my purpose in suing was to understand what really happened to Thomas in that hospital and to make the doctors accountable. So the amount Elizabeth suggested was a big surprise to me.

Elizabeth's closing argument was so passionate—I could not have been more proud to have been represented by her. Win or lose, I knew she was emotionally invested in this case. We were not just another case for her, and that meant the world to me. I took her hand and squeezed it the way she had done for me earlier in the trial, and we shared a tight-lipped but genuine smile as we both fought back more tears.

Mr. Fowler then took the floor.

"This case started and ended with a lot of emotion. Your jury instructions will say that you shouldn't let emotion of any type enter into your deliberative process. This is an important decision to change the life of Dr. Chad. We understand there is a number here that they want to hit. They want a newspaper article at the end of the day."

Elizabeth objected. "That's an inflammatory statement."

The judge overruled her. Mr. Fowler continued.

"What the court wants, what the rules require, is a cold, logical analysis of the facts of the case, and those facts show that you've not been getting the whole truth—that every time you got snippets, you got little portions of testimony, little bits of medical records taken out of context to support a very guided and purposeful theory.

"Their theory in this case is easy. The man was fine. He was well, he was active up until the next to last day, and that the only thing that killed him was a GI bleed. That's the theory, and somehow all these doctors couldn't figure it out. And Dr. Chad is responsible because he didn't do one thing—he didn't give the platelets, and if he'd just ordered these platelets, that would have changed the outcome of this case."

Mr. Fowler's sarcasm was so thick it was unpalatable. I wanted to cover my ears until he was done.

"But did they play the GI doctor's complete testimony? They didn't do that in their case. They played a short video clip where they asked him specifically about the platelets. But what did he say when we played the entire clip? He said it wasn't any one thing. He talked about how all of the issues—the sepsis, the kidney failure, all of it—had to be resolved before he could do an endoscopy. And if Mr. Brown had died during that time period, would there be a question today as to whether or not the GI doctor deviated from the standard of care, taking an unstable patient and doing an endoscopy that could cause him to die? He did the appropriate thing, which was to wait until Mr. Brown was stable. There was nothing to be done to help salvage him in any way, shape, or form because, ladies and gentlemen, it was a multi-organ failure that caused Mr. Brown's death.

"They are saying this was an intentional act. Dr. Chad knew he could save him, and he convinced Mrs. Brown and tricked her into taking her husband to hospice? Think about how that sounds. That is *not* the evidence."

From there, Mr. Fowler proceeded to attack each and every witness with an arrogance that was infuriating. He attempted to show that our experts' testimony and the facts of the case were something other than what we presented.

"Can you judge someone's credibility? That's one of your jobs—looking at him, evaluating Dr. Chad, to figure out if this is the kind of guy who would literally let a healthy guy die of a GI bleed and then tell the wife he needs hospice. Does anyone think that would be the case?

"We know Mrs. Brown admits she wanted to sue for medical malpractice immediately after he died. The question is, was there an agenda from that first moment? You heard from Mrs. Brown that she had a loving relationship with her husband. There was no doubt, ladies and gentlemen, that was the case. She's a sympathetic witness, and she should be. She's a strong, educated woman who likes control."

He's just so nasty, sarcastic, and sexist, I thought.

"She admitted that she did not like this outcome. She was angry at her husband's illness. And she claimed only Dr. Chad told her about the poor prognosis. But you remember, ladies and gentlemen, that there was another doctor that she didn't like very much who on the twenty-seventh said something to her—Dr. Zeller. He told her he'd seen this before and that Mr. Brown would probably not live because he had multi-organ failure.

"I believe Mrs. Brown was angry at the system. She's angry at everything, and there's nothing we're going to be able to do to try to tell her we did everything appropriately. We ask you to remain logical in your analysis of this case and make your decision based on facts, not emotion. We believe the evidence is clear, and if you keep your mind clear, you will see logic in this case."

Oh, now he's playing the race card, I thought. *I'm the angry Black woman. Everyone now knows that something went terribly wrong with my husband's care, but he's attacking me to do anything to win.*

"After I sit down, the plaintiff's attorney will have a short period of time in which to rebut things. I'm not allowed up a second time, but she is because they have the burden of proof."

Mr. Fowler thanked the jury for their time, and Elizabeth stood for her rebuttal. She pointed out that the defense did not even bring Dr. Hamilton in to testify, that they were essentially hiding him from her and the jury and asked why an organization with nothing to hide would do that. She then pointed out that if they could not defend the medicine, then the tactic would be to attack the attorney on the other side, the experts on the other side, and then finally, the woman who brought the case. She took them to task for disparaging me as angry and characterizing me as being financially motivated.

Then Elizabeth pointed out a glaring contradiction in the defense's closing argument—the claim that Thomas died of multi-organ failure. Elizabeth reminded the jury that in none of the medical records was there any indication of multi-organ failure, including the autopsy report, and challenged them to find it in the records that they would be allowed to review during deliberation.

Finally, Elizabeth said, "Take a look at the quote over the judge's head. It says, 'Equal justice under the law.' That's all we want. The judge will not ever give you any instructions that say you cannot be human. This is a civil trial. We can't just say, 'Oh, things happen, there's nothing you can do.' I say it's America, and that's not true. We have a jury system, and we can say this shouldn't have happened.

"Mrs. Brown didn't come to you for sympathy. She came to you for justice. We have every hope and faith in you that you will make a decision in our case—and we will live with it, no matter what it is. We trust you. Thank you."

Elizabeth came back and sat down next to me. I could see that she was drained. She had put her heart and soul into this case and into her closing argument.

* * *

We waited in the courtroom while the jury deliberated.

After a couple of hours passed, Elizabeth knew the deliberations were not going the way she anticipated. She sat down next to me.

"At least someone is fighting for us," she said, referring to someone on the jury.

"Yeah," I said. "And somebody is fighting for the other side too."

"You know," I continued. "I never really expected this court to serve me. I never did. I was hoping it would, but the system was never intended to serve me." Elizabeth just looked at me. "I'm a Black person sitting here with mostly white people around me. Old, rich, white men defending against me, saying all these things, calling me angry, accusing me of being financially motivated. This system isn't going to work for me. It was never intended to."

Elizabeth nodded but said nothing. What could she say?

After a while, Elizabeth said she was going to retry this case and asked what I thought. She was already assuming that we would not receive a guilty verdict. Of course, I said, "Absolutely." I was not going to let this potential setback stop me from making this hospital and these doctors accountable for what they did to Thomas. Elizabeth began discussing her thoughts of how to approach this case the second time around.

We talked a bit more, then headed outside the courtroom because deliberations were taking quite a long time. After a while longer, around 6:00 p.m., the bailiff called us back in. The jury had sent a note to the judge.

They were deadlocked.

The judge called for the jury to come back to the courtroom. "I know all of you have worked hard to try to find a verdict in this case," she said. "But there should be no disagreements about the law. That's my problem, not yours. If you disagree over what you believe the evidence shows, only you can resolve that conflict.

"I only have one request of you. By law, I cannot demand this of you. I want you to go back into the jury room. Taking turns, tell each of the jurors about any weaknesses of your own position. You should not interrupt each other or comment on each other's views. When each of you has stated your case, if you simply cannot reach a verdict, then return to the courtroom. I will declare this case to be a mistrial, and you will be discharged with our appreciation. You will now retire to continue your deliberations."

* * *

After a short while, the jury returned. They were still deadlocked. The judge declared a mistrial and dismissed the jurors.

The judge then told us that it was fair to say that she would not be the judge on the case again and that it would go back to the docket of Judge Weiss, the judge who was supposed to be on the case in the first place and made the decisions on the motions in limine. She stated that if he was like any other judge that it was going to be a year at the very least before we could get another trial date because of the amount of time it took to try the case. Additionally, Judge Weiss no longer had a backup judge to assist him.

"It's not good news for either of your clients," she said. "So, I think this would be an opportunity to settle this case. I take from the jury's notes that it sounds like they were divided. Next time, it's going to be harder and longer. I think you ought to take a really hard look at getting this painful case settled. I suggest that you not bring this case back to court and take up additional court resources. Good luck to all of you. I enjoyed working with you, and I wish you all the best."

Dismissed, we walked out of the courthouse in silence.

* * *

A few months after Thomas's death, before I made the decision to sue Viewpark Hospital and its doctors, I researched medical malpractice lawsuits and the probability of winning my case. A 2016 comprehensive study by Johns Hopkins researchers of medical errors in the US found that an average of 250,000 people in the US die because of medical mistakes each year.[1] That means that medical malpractice is the third leading cause of death, behind cancer and cardiovascular diseases.

Interestingly, only about 2 percent of the patients or their families file a malpractice claim—about 5,000 claims. Of those that file a medical malpractice lawsuit, only 7 percent or 350 of the lawsuits end in a trial, as many cases are either dropped or dismissed before trial. And of that amount that go to trial, only about 5 percent of them, or 18 cases, end in a verdict, and 95 percent, or 332 cases, end with an out-of-court

---

1   Martin Makary and Michael Daniel, "Medical Error—the Third Leading Cause of Death in the US," *BMJ* 2016, no. 353 (2016): i2139, https://doi.org/10.1136/bmj.i2139.

settlement.[2] Accordingly, I always knew that the chances of winning my case at trial were slim.

* * *

A few days after the end of the trial, two of the jurors independently called Elizabeth. Hank, the jury foreman, and Tammy were both troubled by the mistrial and wanted to speak with Elizabeth further about it. Both of them told her nearly identical stories.

It seemed that at the beginning of deliberations, a vote was taken of the six jurors. Hank and Tammy believed that this initial vote would be six to none, in our favor. They were shocked to find, even in light of all the compelling evidence, that there were two who believed otherwise. The four jurors in our favor made a serious effort to present piece after piece of evidence to convince the two holdouts that the evidence was clear that the hospital and doctors were negligent.

But there was nothing that could be said to sway the two holdouts to consider a different viewpoint, although they offered up no real evidence to support their position. One of the two seemed to be the more forceful in her opposition to a verdict in our favor, while the other juror had little to say but supported the other opposing juror anyway.

Hank and Tammy went on to tell Elizabeth that these two opposing jurors even crossed their arms and would not participate in the exercise that the judge requested of all of them. Although the judge could not require it of the jurors, she wanted each of them to discuss the weakness in their own position. They refused to do so.

---

2 "US Medical Malpractice Case Statistics," Justpoint, accessed March 22, 2023, https://justpoint.com/knowledge-base/us-medical-malpractice-case-statistics/.

Hank and Tammy both told Elizabeth that she had done a great job of presenting my case. The expert testimonies were excellent. The way the evidence was presented was clear. They apologized for not being able to bring all of the jurors together for a win for our side.

When I asked Elizabeth what her opinion was as to why we lost the case when it was so strong, she shared these jurors' conversations with me.

"We got a hung jury in this case," she said, "because one woman did not want to find against the doctor and another woman sided with her. This is not something we'll ever figure out because we don't know this one woman or what she was thinking. What we *do* know is the two women didn't have any factual reasons for finding against us. One woman was against us for reasons we'll never know—and for whatever reason, she brought the other lady along with her. I don't think it has anything to do with the facts and strength of our case or the way we presented it, because you're right—we should've won this case easily. Jury selection is a crapshoot, and somehow, we guessed wrong on this one woman.

"I'm sorry, Jonnie."

MY PROMISE

IN JANUARY OF 2020, ELIZABETH CALLED ME.

"Jonnie," she said, "I'm going after the GI doctor. I'm going to sue him by himself."

I had to get justice for Thomas, so I told her I was glad to hear this. She called back a few days later.

"I heard from his attorney, and they're fighting me all the way to court. I told him, fine, let's go to court, because now you won't have just me fighting you—you're going to have the other party fighting you too, trying to blame everything on you. So, we'll all go to court."

Elizabeth talked to the GI doctor's attorney on a few more occasions, and she told me she could tell he was weakening. Finally, they called her back and asked why *did* the hospital send Thomas to hospice when their client could have done the surgery—the same question we had been asking from the outset. They saw what we saw and decided the fight was not worth it.

This was in March of 2020, right when coronavirus was hitting the national news and the country was shutting down. I thought about how the defense dwelled on the RSV during the trial, and I sent a text message to Elizabeth, expressing my concern that when we retry our case, jurors might get confused about the coronavirus, causing thousands of deaths at the time, versus the RSV infection.

Elizabeth called me immediately to tell me she shared my concern about not only that, but also about the fact that the courts were shut down due to the pandemic, which threatened to push out our case even further than the year the judge had predicted. In addition, potential jurors were likely going to be sympathetic to medical personnel—as they should be—considering everything they were going through battling COVID-19. Even if we were able to win—to get a six-person jury to find in our favor—the losing party would automatically appeal, trying to find errors in law or procedures at trial significant enough to overturn the verdict. That could take another year. It could be four or five years before we saw any damages, provided we overcame all of these obstacles.

So, she recommended I settle.

I reminded Elizabeth that I was willing to settle for a fair amount before the trial began and that it was the hospital that wanted to go to court, so I did not mind reconsidering that option. Elizabeth immediately started negotiations and texted me about her every step.

When the settlement amount offered was one that Elizabeth and I found acceptable, Elizabeth settled. She emailed me the nondisclosure documents, along with closing statements, and indicated where I should sign.

I sat on the paperwork for a few days. I had no sense of satisfaction, and I asked myself, *Why?*

I never expected money to comfort me for losing Thomas. That could never happen. I did not know what I would feel when the settlement was negotiated, but I was not satisfied because the people who did not provide Thomas with the proper care did not pay any real price. The insurance companies would pay Elizabeth and me; the doctors would not. These doctors were free to do to others exactly what they had done to Thomas. They could go home every evening to enjoy their families, while my family was destroyed and I am now alone every day.

I called Elizabeth to ask if the settlements stopped me from telling people what happened.

"Is this story still mine?" I asked her.

"This story is still yours," she said.

"I can write a book about this?"

"You can write a book about this."

The next thing I wanted to know was whether or not the settlement prohibited me from filing complaints with the Florida Licensing and Regulation Board. Elizabeth told me I could do that too.

"But you're not going to win," she said.

"Why can't I win?"

"Because the agency is not sufficiently funded, and they don't have the resources to properly investigate the medical complaints that are received," Elizabeth said.

I thought for a moment. "But my complaint will be accepted, right?"

"Yes."

"Will the doctor or the hospital be notified that I filed a complaint?"

"Yes."

"They must respond to my complaint, right?"

"Yes."

"And a notification of the findings of the investigation will eventually be sent out?"

"Yes."

"Then if that's the best I can hope for from this so-called oversight agency, so be it. These doctors *have* to account for their negligent actions somehow. I want the responsible parties to have to spend time responding to my complaint—to defend their licenses, to worry about a mark on their professional record, to hopefully reflect on what they could have done differently to save a life, and to never underestimate another family again." I paused. "Maybe my complaint will be the very thing to make them provide better care to avoid a future complaint. Maybe—just maybe, they will be more careful before they hurt another family."

"It might be helpful, dear," Elizabeth said, "if you indicate in your complaint that I have all the medical records, depositions, transcripts of the trials, the autopsy report, and any other documentation they may require for their investigation. I'm happy to allow them access to all of my records."

"Thank you, Elizabeth. That is so kind of you. That would certainly make it easier for the board to investigate my complaints, if they find the means to do so."

I ran into a few challenges when trying to get the settlement papers notarized because so many businesses had limited appointments or were closed down due to COVID-19, and because of the requirement for two witnesses. But I eventually obtained all of the proper signatures and sent the papers back to Elizabeth for further handling.

* * *

I wanted to hear firsthand Hank's and Tammy's comments and observations about the trial, so Elizabeth arranged for me to speak with them directly. In addition, Frances—the Black nurse who cared for Thomas when he was abandoned in unofficial ICU—had coincidentally contacted Elizabeth for her own personal matter. Elizabeth recognized her name and put us in touch with one another. Most significant, I subsequently had a more in-depth conversation with Elizabeth.

I prepared a set of questions beforehand so everyone would have an idea of what I was going to ask. I spoke to Hank, Tammy, Frances, and Elizabeth separately via Zoom for about two hours each.

Hank works in the information technology field, and I immediately got a sense of his strong analytical and organizational skills. No wonder he was selected as the foreman. Tammy worked in the accounting field early in her career but has since been a caretaker for several different family members. She is obviously the backbone of her family and is most proud of her thirty-two years of marriage.

Hank and Tammy were pretty much in sync with each other about the merits of my case. They both thought Dr. Hamilton was trying to hide since he did not show up in court and his name was seldom mentioned. They both believed that finding in my favor would send a message to the doctors and the hospital that policy and procedural changes were necessary so that a situation like mine would not happen again.

They also both stated that ageism played a part in the jury's delibera-tions. One of the opposing jurors said that Thomas had a lot of things wrong with him and that he was going to die anyway, so it did not matter that the endoscopy was never done. She was young and did not seem to understand that the conditions Thomas had prior to this hospital encounter were manageable and ones that people live with everyday.

Hank systematically evaluated the case, comparing what was happen-ing *to* Thomas to what was being done *for* Thomas. He concluded that Dr. Chad was not well organized or competent; he did not own his responsibility to ensure that proper care was provided, and he did not follow through to the best of his ability to achieve a favorable outcome for his patient. Hank found it amazing that all the doctors did not talk to each other and relied on notes that were not completed during the day, especially given that the notes were in English, even though English was not the first language of several of the doctors.

Hank also noted that he would have liked subtitles for the videos, since some witnesses had thick accents. He didn't know at the time that the defense argued against subtitles and won. He would have liked more time to review videos and other evidence, but time ran out because the evidence had not been digitized so that searches could be quickly performed. Finally, Hank was disappointed in the brevity of the autopsy report but found out after the trial that the full report was not made available to the jurors.

Tammy said the case was clinched for her when one of the defense's witnesses, Dr. Barber from Florida, clearly stated that the platelets were too valuable for Thomas and that they should be saved for the trauma unit. *Why wasn't Thomas's critical condition worthy of the plate-lets?* Tammy wondered. Platelets are only good for a certain amount of time so they should not be held, anticipating a situation that may not occur. Tammy also could not understand why Thomas was not placed in ICU considering his grave condition.

Tammy was very impressed with my son, Michael, as he was very professional, calm, and well-spoken. When leaving the courtroom after the mistrial was declared, she could not look Michael in the eye because she felt she had let us down. Tammy could not sleep for the first couple of nights following the end of the trial. She told Elizabeth to keep her phone number, as this case is part of her life now and she wants to know how things work out for me. Since being a juror on this case, Tammy has become a platelet donor.

My discussion with Frances was also quite revealing. She chose to become a nurse because her mother had medical issues and she wanted to be able to properly care for her. As a contractor, she usually does not work on Sundays, but because she needed more hours that week, she accepted this assignment for the Sunday that Thomas was left alone.

Frances said that a patient should never be handed off to the next shift when they are dirty like Thomas was on that morning. He should not have been left lying in those bloody stools because it is bad for the skin. She also said that seventy-four is not old and Thomas should have been given the best of care, regardless of his age. Frances said that you could not pay her to see the GI doctor that was consulted for Thomas's condition. Apparently he is wealthy and does not need the work nor the money, so he generally shows little interest in his patients.

Frances is sympathetic to patients who only have Medicare. The Viewpark Hospital doctors usually do not order all of the tests that may be necessary to diagnose a patient's condition, and she wonders how many people have lost their lives or do not get the care they need because of their insurance.

In her past assignments at Viewpark, Frances experienced several misunderstandings in instructions received regarding patient care and her work schedule. She also observed on several occasions substandard

treatment for Black patients as compared to white patients—in particular, addressing patient pain. Some doctors believe that Black people
do not experience pain like other patients, so they will give a lower
dose of medication to Black patients or will even send Black patients
home in pain, telling them to see a pain specialist.

Frances continued, saying that doctors at Viewpark speak to Black
patients differently than white patients and for a shorter length of
time. In addition, Black patients and their families are often reluctant
to ask questions, and when they do, the doctors do not like it and are
not as forthcoming with answers—just like my experience. In short,
Frances told me Viewpark Hospital failed me. She advised me to know
the Patient's Bill of Rights for future encounters with the medical
profession.

Finally, I really appreciated the time Elizabeth gave me to ask her
additional questions about my case. She said that she conducted six
or seven focus groups to consider my case. A focus group is a research
method that allows attorneys to explore the attitudes of individuals
who are demographically representative of the people who may be in
our jury pool. Every one of Elizabeth's focus groups found in my favor
and suggested a range of amounts that she should ask for in court for
damages. Focus groups, as we experienced, cannot predict the outcome
of the actual trial case.

Elizabeth was quite upset when a mistrial was declared because this
case is the worst medical malpractice case she has ever seen in her
forty years of practice. She cannot get over the fact that Thomas did
not come to the hospital with a bleeding ulcer, that he was neglected
long enough that he died. Most of her cases involved an emergency
situation where mistakes were made because decisions about care had
to be made very quickly. This case was not an emergency; it required a
simple fix, and there was plenty of time to fix it.

Elizabeth made it clear that the purpose of tort law is to improve the standard of medical care for patients. Most people do not sue because they do not understand the patient's issues and they do not know enough about the quality of the care received. Doctors are often gracious and sympathetic, saying "I'm sorry" so many patients and their families accept the outcome without question. Doctors usually try to display a good bedside manner while all doctors and nurses protect one another, making it difficult to learn that something went amiss. She pointed out that I, too, did not know enough about what happened with Thomas's care at Viewpark Hospital. The difference, however, was that I knew Thomas was not seriously ill when he entered the hospital.

I am forever grateful to have found Elizabeth as my attorney. Everyone on her team was completely committed to me and united in their efforts to put on the best case for me. By all measures, we should have won my case.

* * *

A couple of months following the settlements with the GI doctor and the hospital, I researched recent complaints that may have been filed against Viewpark Hospital. The only information I could find were several billing complaints filed with the Better Business Bureau. I asked Elizabeth to forward me the copies of the hospital billings to BCBS and Medicare, since Viewpark Hospital never sent me a detailed billing of all hospital charges. When I received them, I saw—as an ex-auditor—what I thought I might see.

It appears that Viewpark Hospital billed my insurance company and Medicare expensive ICU rates for the time Thomas was lying in *unofficial* ICU, receiving inadequate medical care and being left unattended in his own filth.

* * *

Every day, I cannot help but think about the American institutions that failed Thomas and me when we needed them the most—the healthcare delivery system, the legal system, and most likely, the medical quality assurance system of Florida. I thought that telling my husband's personal story could impact this long legacy of discrimination and abuse against African Americans in the healthcare system. Thomas's story must bring more awareness to the fact that racism, including implicit bias, remains the root cause of continued disparities in death and disease between Black and white people in the United States today. Academic and governmental studies support these findings.

As a nation, we must understand that the roots of today's health disparities lie in slavery. One of the many cruelties that Black people suffered during that legalized and inhumane institution was lack of healthcare, laying the groundwork for today's health disparities. During slavery and throughout our nation's history, people of color have been the subject of terrifying medical research and experimentation while white physicians and institutions have become wealthy and celebrated. For instance, clinical scientists experimented with Henrietta Lacks's cells without her family's permission, resulting in many medical breakthroughs and two Nobel prizes for the scientists.

In the Tuskegee Study, US government researchers withheld syphilis treatment from Black men, observing them until they died. The families of the participants won a $10 million class action settlement in 1975 and an apology from President Bill Clinton in 1997. This is one of the most notorious examples from an exhaustive list that demonstrates how Black people have been betrayed by the medical establishment.

Most disgraceful is that nearly 160 years after legalized slavery was abolished, health inequities between Black and white Americans still exist, in spite of our "contributions" to medicine. Slavery ended, but myths used to justify slavery remain embedded in our culture, our minds, and our souls. Many of these myths—for example, Black people are not as sensitive to physical and emotional pain as white people—are still believed by some physicians today. We must ask ourselves, *Why?*

What will it take for this nation to do some soul searching to understand, acknowledge, and address our biases?

What will it take for Black bodies to be respected by the medical profession and other American institutions?

Racism touches every aspect of Black people's lives. For my family, it has culminated with the untimely and unnecessary death of my husband at the hands of those who created life-threatening conditions where there were none, when they could have used their knowledge and power to save his life. Healthcare professionals must commit to undoing centuries of hurt and harm and fight for adequate healthcare for all. Some universities, professional organizations, and governmental entities are developing strategies to address this subject, but progress has not come soon enough for my family.

Patients call on the medical profession when they are at their most vulnerable, when they are uncertain and worried because they are unwell. Imagine adding to that the fear and stress associated with wondering if their treatment will be adequate or not, based on the color of their skin. Patients must know that they have the right and the means to report mistreatment and unethical behavior. Know and understand the Patient's Bill of Rights. File a complaint with the state health department about the facility; or the state licensing board for specific providers; or the accreditation commission for hospitals; or the US Department of Health and Human Services, Office of Civil Rights, for discrimination; or the designated agency in a particular jurisdiction. Sue in civil court. When patients and their families consistently take action when warranted, it may become a deterrent to discrimination and inadequate healthcare occurring in the first place.

I refuse to let institutions and persons with distorted views that include racism and ageism dictate to me that Thomas and I do not matter. I wrote this book in an effort to fight every day for justice for my husband—that gentleman and gentle man—who did not deserve to be neglected and mistreated in that Florida hospital. This is my effort to turn my emotional pain and anguish into purpose, hoping that sharing our experience can make a positive difference in someone else's life, be it patient or practitioner. As my family's historian, I will tell Thomas's story for the rest of my life so generations will know what really happened to Thomas and me and how we tried to make a difference for others.

That is *my* promise.

ACKNOWLEDGMENTS

To my husband, Thomas James Brown: every day, from the moment we met, you loved me with your mind, body, and soul. Because of this, I knew I could not rest until I told your story and let everyone know what an extraordinary man you were.

This book came together with exceptional support from the very talented Kathleen McIntosh and John Vercher, my editors extraordinaire, who I appreciate beyond measure. Thank you also to Rikki Jump, Sophie May, Kacy Wren, Anna Dorfman, and all the others at Scribe Media.

Special thanks goes to Elizabeth Faiella, my Florida attorney, who believed in my case from the start, and her team, Peter, Becki, Janice, Jill, and Amanda. Thank you for giving your all to a case we should have won, taking care of me at this very painful time in my life, and encouraging me before, during, and after the court trial.

Thank you to my family and friends, especially Thomasine Greer, Michael and Marna Marsh, and Martha "Cookie" Lyons, who supported me throughout Thomas's ordeal when he was hospitalized and then bore witness in court. I know I can always depend on them whenever I am in need. Also, there are many other special people, too many to mention, who listened and provided counsel or other assistance throughout the process of writing this book. They know who they are, and I am extremely grateful to all of them.

Last, but never least, I am thankful to my mother and father, the late Catherine and Alfred Ramsey, who were always there for me. They helped raise my son, especially in his early years while I was working full time during the day and attending college in the evening to create a better life. They were supportive in every possible way they knew how.

REFERENCES
AND READINGS

African Americans have historically faced discrimination and abuse by medical professionals in the United States, as documented by innumerable medical studies and frequent coverage in the news. In fact, over eighty-four thousand Black and brown lives are needlessly lost each year as a result of unconscious racial and ethnic biases.[3] To combat these disparities, advocates say healthcare professionals must explicitly acknowledge and examine how race and racism factor into healthcare and how equally effective treatment can be provided for all persons in the United States.

The following is a partial list of books and online articles that discuss healthcare disparities for African Americans in the United States and how this second-rate healthcare is shortening lives.

---

3 Matthew, *Just Medicine.*

BOOKS

Barr, Donald A. *Health Disparities in the United States: Social Class, Race, Ethnicity and the Social Determinants of Health.* Baltimore: Johns Hopkins University Press, 2019.

Bridges, Khiara M. *Critical Race Theory: A Primer (Concepts and Insights).* St. Paul, MN: Foundation Press, 2018.

Chanoff, David, and Louis W. Sullivan. *We'll Fight It Out Here: A History of the Ongoing Struggle for Health Equity.* Baltimore: Johns Hopkins University Press, 2022.

Hannah-Jones, Nikole, Cairtlin Roper, Ilena Silverman, and Jake Silverstein, eds. *The 1619 Project: A New Origin Story.* New York: One World, 2021.

Hoberman, John. *Black and Blue: The Origins and Consequences of Medical Racism.* Los Angeles: University of California Press, 2012.

LaVeist, Thomas A., and Lydia A. Isaac, eds. *Race, Ethnicity, and Health: A Public Reader.* 2nd ed. San Francisco: Jossey-Bass, 2013.

Matthew, Dayna Bowen. *Just Health: Treating Structural Racism to Heal America.* New York: New York University Press, 2022.

Matthew, Dayna Bowen. *Just Medicine: A Cure for Racial Inequality in American Health Care.* New York: New York University Press, 2018.

Oparah, Julia Chinyere, Helen Arega, Dantia Hudson, Linda Jones, and Talita Oseguera. *Battling over Birth: Black Women and the Maternal Health Care Crisis.* Amarillo, TX: Praeclarus Press, 2018.

Satcher, David. *My Quest for Health Equity: Notes on Learning While Leading*. Baltimore: Johns Hopkins University Press, 2020.

Tweedy, Damon. *Black Man in a White Coat: A Doctor's Reflections on Race and Medicine*. New York: Picador, 2015.

Villarosa, Linda. *Under The Skin: The Hidden Toll of Racism on American Lives and on the Health of Our Nation*. New York: Doubleday, 2022.

Washington, Harriett A. *Medical Apartheid: The Dark History of Medical Experimentation on Black Americans from Colonial Times to the Present*. New York: Harlem Moon, 2006.

ONLINE ARTICLES

Alcindor, Yamiche, Rachel Wellford, Bria Lloyd, and Lizz Bolaji. "With a History of Abuse in American Medicine, Black Patients Struggle for Equal Access." *PBS*, February 24, 2021. https://www.pbs.org/newshour/show/with-a-history-of-abuse-in-american-medicine-black-patients-struggle-for-equal-access.

American Patients Rights Association. "AHA Patient's Bill of Rights." Accessed March 22, 2023. https://www.americanpatient.org/aha-patients-bill-of-rights/.

Anderson, Javonte. "America Has a History of Medically Abusing Black People. No Wonder Many Are Wary of Covid-19 Vaccines." *USA Today*, March 3, 2021. https://www.usatoday.com/story/news/2021/02/16/black-history-covid-vaccine-fears-medical-experiments/4358844001/.

Asare, Janice Gassam. "How One Woman's Story of Medical Neglect Highlights the Pervasive Issue of Racism in Healthcare." *Forbes*, July 2,

2021. https://www.forbes.com/sites/janicegassam/2021/07/02/
how-one-womans-story-of-medical-neglect-highlights-the-perva-
sive-issue-of-racism-in-healthcare/?sh=1fca7b01270b.

Balch, Bridgett. "Racism—Not Race—Drives Health Disparities." AAMC.
November 13, 2022. https://www.aamc.org/news-insights/racism-
not-race-drives-health-disparities.

Boden, Sarah. "A New Hippocratic Oath Asks Doctors to Fight Racial Injustice and Misinformation." Shots, NPR. November 4, 2020. https://
www.npr.org/sections/health-shots/2020/11/04/929233492/a-
new-hippocratic-oath-asks-doctors-to-fight-racial-injustice-and-
misinformation.

Boehmer, Tegan K., Emily H. Koumans, Elizabeth L. Skillen, Michael D.
Kappelman, Thomas W. Carton, Aditiben Patel, Euna M. August
et al. "Racial and Ethnic Disparities in Outpatient Treatment of
COVID-19—United States, January–July 2022." *Morbidity and
Mortality Weekly Report* 71, no. 43 (October 28, 2022): 1359–65.
http://dx.doi.org/10.15585/mmwr.mm7143a2.

Bridges, Khiara M. "Implicit Bias and Racial Disparities in Health Care."
Human Rights Magazine 43, no. 3 (August 2018). https://www.
americanbar.org/groups/crsj/publications/human_rights_mag-
azine_home/the-state-of-healthcare-in-the-united-states/ra-
cial-disparities-in-health-care/.

Burgess, Diana J. "Are Providers More Likely to Contribute to Healthcare
Disparities under High Levels of Cognitive Load? How Features
of the Healthcare Setting May Lead to Biases in Medical Decision
Making." *Medical Decision Making* 30, no. 2 (2010): 246–57. https://
doi.org/10.1177/0272989X09341751.

Caraballo, César, Daisy S. Massey, Chima D. Ndumele, Trent Haywood, Shayaan Kaleem, Terris King, Yuntian Liu, et al. "Excess Mortality and Years of Potential Life Lost among the Black Population in the US, 1999–2020." JAMA 329, no. 19 (2023): 1662–70. https://doi. org/10.1001/jama.2023.7022.

Chu, Edward, and Kenneth Igbalode. "Feature: Black Lives Need to Matter: Examining the Inequalities Within Medicine." *Cardiology Magazine*, American College of Cardiology. June 11, 2020. https:// www.acc.org/latest-in-cardiology/articles/2020/06/01/12/42/ feature-black-lives-need-to-matter-examining-the-inequalities-within-medicine.

Colarossi, Jessica. "Why Black Women Face More Health Risks Before, During, and After Pregnancy: Researchers at Boston University Are Working to Eliminate Racial Disparities in Maternal Health." The Brink, Boston University. October 29, 2019. http://www.bu.edu/articles/2019/racial-disparities-in-maternal-health/.

Coombs, Bertha. "Black Doctors Push for Anti-Bias Training in Medicine to Combat Health Inequality." *CNBC*, June 10, 2020. https://www. cnbc.com/2020/06/19/black-doctors-prescription-for-changing-racial-inequity-in-health-care.html.

Ejiofor, Annette. "Serena Williams: U.S. Doctors Are Failing Black Women during Childbirth." *HuffPost*, March 7, 2018. https://www.huffingtonpost.ca/2018/03/07/serena-williams-doctors-black-women_a_23379506/.

Gomez, Alan, Wyatte Grantham-Philips, Trevor Hughes, Rick Jervis, Rebecca Plevin, Kameel Stanley, Dennis Wagner, Marco della Cava, Deborah Barfield Berry, and Mark Nichols. "'An Unbelievable Chain of Oppression': America's History of Racism Was a Pre-Existing Condition for COVID-19." *USA Today*, October 21, 2020. https://www.usatoday.com/in-depth/news/nation/2020/10/12/coronavirus-deaths-reveal-systemic-racism-united-states/5770952002/.

Helm, Angela. "Kira Johnson Spoke 5 Languages, Raced Cars, Was Daughter-in-Law of Judge Glenda Hackett. She Still Died in Childbirth." *The Root*, October 19, 2018. https://www.theroot.com/kira-johnson-spoke-5-languages-raced-cars-was-daughte-1829862323.

Holland, Brynn. "The 'Father of Modern Gynecology' Performed Shocking Experiments on Enslaved Women." History.com. December 4, 2018. https://www.history.com/news/the-father-of-modern-gynecology-performed-shocking-experiments-on-slaves.

Hostetter, Martha, and Sarah Klein. "In Focus: Reducing Racial Disparities in Health Care by Confronting Racism." The Commonwealth Fund. September 27, 2018. https://www.commonwealthfund.org/publications/2018/sep/focus-reducing-racial-disparities-health-care-confronting-racism.

Huerto, Ryan. "Minority Patients Benefit from Having Minority Doctors, but That's a Hard Match to Make." *Health Lab* (blog), Michigan Medicine, University of Michigan. March 31, 2020. https://labblog.uofmhealth.org/rounds/minority-patients-benefit-from-having-minority-doctors-but-thats-a-hard-match-to-make-0.

Imhoff, Jordyn. "Health Inequality Actually Is a Black and White Issue, Research Says: A Roundup of 10 Studies Highlighting the Health Disparities between Black and White Americans." *Health Lab* (blog), Michigan Medicine, University of Michigan. June 3, 2020. https://healthblog.uofmhealth.org/lifestyle/health-inequality-actually-a-black-and-white-issue-research-says.

Jalloh, Abubakarr. "How the Pandemic's Unequal Toll on People of Color Underlines US Health Inequities—and Why Solving Them Is So Critical." The Conversation. January 19, 2022. https://theconversation. com/how-the-pandemics-unequal-toll-on-people-of-color-underlines-us-health-inequities-and-why-solving-them-is-so-critical-169151.

Jones, Nancy L. "Structural Racism and Health Inequities in the USA: Evidence and Interventions." *American Journal of Public Health* 110, no. 9 (September 2020): 1258–59. https://doi.org/10.2105/ AJPH.2020.305823.

Kyere, Eric. "Enslaved People's Health Was Ignored from the Country's Beginning, Laying the Groundwork for Today's Health Disparities." The Conversation. July 30, 2020. https://theconversation. com/enslaved-peoples-health-was-ignored-from-the-countrys-beginning-laying-the-groundwork-for-todays-health-disparities-143339.

Lawson, Marissa, and Christoph Lee. "Biopsies Confirm a Breast Cancer Diagnosis after an Abnormal Mammogram—but Structural Racism May Lead to Lengthy Delays." The Conversation. July 8, 2022. https://theconversation.com/biopsies-confirm-a-breast-cancer-diagnosis-after-an-abnormal-mammogram-but-structural-racism-may-lead-to-lengthy-delays-185824.

Ledbetter, Carly. "Serena Williams: 'Doctors Aren't Listening So Black Women Are Dying.'" *HuffPost*, March 9, 2018. https://www.huffpost.com/ entry/serena-williams-black-women-health-care_n_5aa156fce4b002df2c61c6aa.

Mandal, Ananya. "Ending Health Disparities." News Medical. Last updated February 26, 2019. https://www.news-medical.net/health/Ending-Health-Disparities.aspx.

Mandara, James L. "Reckoning with Medicine's History of Racism." AMA. February 17, 2021. https://www.ama-assn.org/about/leadership/reckoning-medicine-s-history-racism.

Miliano, Brett. "How Slavery Still Shadows Healthcare." *The Harvard Gazette,* October 29, 2019. https://news.harvard.edu/gazette//story/2019/10/ramifications-of-slavery-persist-in-health-care-in-equality/.

Nirappil, Fenit. "A Black Doctor Alleged Racist Treatment before Dying of Covid-19: 'This Is How Black People Get Killed'." *Washington Post,* December 24, 2020. https://www.washingtonpost.com/health/2020/12/24/covid-susan-moore-medical-racism/.

Okwerekwu, Jennifer Adaeze. "What Happened When I Talked about What Others Ignored—Racism in Medicine." STAT. April 27, 2016. https://www.statnews.com/2016/04/27/racism-medicine-lessons/.

Picheta, Rob. "Black Newborns More Likely to Die When Looked After by White Doctors." CNN Health. August 20, 2020. https://www.cnn.com/2020/08/18/health/black-babies-mortality-rate-doctors-study-wellness-scli-intl/index.html.

"Racism and Discrimination in Health Care: Providers and Patients." *Harvard Health Blog,* Harvard Health Publishing, Harvard Medical School. July 9, 2020. https://www.health.harvard.edu/blog/racism-discrimination-health-care-providers-patients-2017011611015.

Smedley, Brian D., Adrienne Y. Stith, and Alan R. Nelson, eds. *Unequal Treatment: Confronting Racial and Ethnic Disparities in Health Care.* Washington, DC: The National Academies Press, 2003. https://doi.org/10.17226/10260.

Smith, Timothy M. "Raced-Based Medicine Is Wrong. How Should Physicians Oppose It?" AMA. December 14, 2020. https://www.ama-assn.org/delivering-care/health-equity/race-based-medicine-wrong-how-should-physicians-oppose-it.

Stallings, Erika. "This Is How the American Healthcare System Is Failing Black Women. Racial Bias Is Real—and It Put These Women's Lives at Risk." Oprah Daily. August 1, 2018. https://www.oprahdaily.com/life/health/a23100351/racial-bias-in-healthcare-black-women/.

Villarosa, Linda. "How False Beliefs in Physical Racial Difference Still Live in Medicine Today." *New York Times Magazine*, August 14, 2019. https://www.nytimes.com/interactive/2019/08/14/magazine/racial-differences-doctors.html

Zaragovia, Verónica. "Trying to Avoid Racist Health Care, Black Women Seek Out Black Obstetricians." Shots, NPR. May 28, 2021. https://www.npr.org/sections/health-shots/2021/05/28/996603360/trying-to-avoid-racist-health-care-black-women-seek-out-black-obstetricians.

ABOUT THE AUTHOR

JONNIE RAMSEY BROWN EARNED HER BACHELOR'S DEGREE IN
1974 and began a career at one of the nation's leading accounting
firms, becoming a Certified Public Accountant. She worked at various
colleges and universities during her career and served on two Olympic organizing committees: Los Angeles in 1984 and Atlanta in 1996. In
2004, she earned her MBA and later became a Certified Information
System Auditor—a cybersecurity professional. Jonnie worked with
the Department of Homeland Security as a System Accountant and,
in 2017, helped FEMA with hurricane disaster relief. She retired from
DHS in 2019.

As her family historian, Jonnie published a compilation of stories
in 2017 about her family and writes articles for various genealogy
publications. She is also a member of the Daughters of the American
Revolution, the Sons and Daughters of the US Middle Passage, First
Families of Alabama, and other lineage, historical, and genealogy organizations. Jonnie now tells her family's personal story to bring awareness to the racial disparities in healthcare, in honor of the legacy of her
late husband, Thomas James Brown.

Made in the USA
Columbia, SC
04 January 2024

29891595R00221